Life After Osteoporosis Diagnosis How to Rebuild Strength and Confidence at Any Age

Sommario

Chapter 1 12

Recognizing Hidden Osteoporosis: You Are Not Your Diagnosis
.... 12

Chapter 2 19

Bone Anatomy and the Remodeling Cycle in Plain English 19

Chapter 3 27

Who Is at Risk and Why: Family, Hormones, Aging 27

Chapter 4 34

Testing Your Bones: DEXA vs TBS and Why Results Change 34

Chapter 5 41

Treatment Choices: Medications, Outcomes, and Non Drug
Paths 41

Chapter 6 49

Food for Strong Bones: How Much Calcium You Need and Best
Foods 49

Chapter 7 56

Supplements Made Simple: D3, K2, Magnesium, Collagen 56

Chapter 8 63

Everyday Safety: How to Avoid Common Fractures at Home and
Outside 63

Chapter 9 70

Posture and Balance: Spine Protection You Can Trust 70

Chapter 10 78

Training that Builds Bone: Principles, Progression, and Realistic Gains 78

Chapter 11 86

Weights, Bands, and Bodyweight: What Works and How Much Load Is Right 86

Chapter 12 93

Walking, Yoga, and Pilates: What Helps, What to Modify, What to Avoid 93

Chapter 13 100

Sports and Hobbies: How to Play Safely and Confidently 100

Chapter 14 108

Lifting Loved Ones: Holding and Carrying Grandchildren Safely 108

Chapter 15 115

Travel with Ease: Planning, Packing, Moving Without Risk 115

Chapter 16 122

Training After a Vertebral Fracture: When You Can Lift Again 122

Chapter 17 129

Decade by Decade: Personalized Bone Care and Weekly Plans 129

Chapter 18 137

Partner with Providers, Debunk Myths, and Live Confidently for Life 137

Sardine & Lemon Kale Toast (Calcium and Protein Rich) 144

Calcium Set Tofu Scramble with Sesame Greens 148

Tahini Chickpea Bowl with Roasted Broccoli and Lemon 152

Baked Salmon Oat Cakes with Lemon Yogurt Sauce 155

Spinach Mushroom Ricotta Frittata (Oven Baked) 159

Cottage Cheese Oat Pancakes with Blueberries 162

White Bean, Kale, and Parmesan Rind Soup 165

Yogurt-Lemon Chicken Thighs with Sesame Broccoli 168

Silken Tofu Berry Smoothie (Dairy Free, Calcium and Protein) ... 171

Ricotta Lemon Stuffed Sweet Potatoes with Garlicky Kale 174

Kefir Overnight Oats with Chia and Almonds 178

Orange Sesame Tofu with Bok Choy (Calcium Set, One Pan) 181

No Bake Almond Tahini Calcium Bites (Travel Friendly Snack) .. 184

Turkey Ricotta Meatballs in Spinach Tomato Sauce 187

Lemon Tahini Lentil Pilaf with Leafy Greens 190

Exercise 1 194

360° Rib Breathing in Tall Sit (Safe Spine Setup) 194

Exercise 2 198

Wall Tall Stand and Head Reach 198

Exercise 3 201

Hip Hinge to Wall Tap 201

Exercise 4 204

Chair Sit to Stand, High Box 204

Exercise 5 207

Hip Hinge Pick Up from 30 cm Platform 207

Exercise 6 210

Supported Single-Leg Stand at Counter 210

Exercise 7 213

Heel-to-Toe Tandem Stand and Walk 213

Exercise 8 216

Head Turns in Single-Leg Stand 216

Exercise 9 219

Step Touch Over Low Line 219

Exercise 10 222

Low Step Up with Rail 222

Exercise 11 225

Mini Band Hip Hinge with Abduction 225

Exercise 12 228

Bridge on Floor, Neutral Spine 228

Exercise 13 231

Supported Split Squat Short Stance 231

Exercise 14 234

Side-Lying Hip Abduction 234

Exercise 15 237

Seated Marches with Neutral Spine 237

Exercise 16 240

Band Row at Chest Height 240

Exercise 17 244

Seated Band Lat Pull to Collarbone 244

Exercise 18 248

Wall Push Up 248

Exercise 19 251

Seated Dumbbell Press to Eye Level 251

Exercise 20 255

Band Chest Press in Split Stance 255

Exercise 21 259

Farmer Carry with Light Dumbbells 259

Exercise 22 263

Suitcase Carry One Side 263

Exercise 23 266

Front Load Carry with Backpack 266

Exercise 24 270

Grocery Bag Lift and Carry Drill 270

Exercise 25 274

Step Down Control from Low Step 274

Exercise 26 277

Dead Bug Heel Taps 277

Exercise 27 280

Side Plank on Knees 280

Exercise 28 283

Pallof Press with Band 283

Exercise 29 286

Bird-Dog Reach Short Range 286

Exercise 30 289

Tall-Kneel Hip Hinge with Dowel 289

Copyright © 2025 by Elena Forti All rights reserved.

No part of this publication may be reproduced, distributed, or transmitted in any form or by any means, including photocopying, recording, or other electronic or mechanical methods, without the prior written permission of the publisher, except in the case of brief quotations used in reviews or articles. This book is intended solely for informational and educational purposes. It does not provide medical advice, diagnosis, or treatment. Readers should always consult their physician or qualified healthcare professional before making any changes to their diet, exercise routine, medication, or treatment plan. The author and publisher disclaim all liability for any injury, loss, or damage allegedly arising from the use or misuse of the information contained in this book. All names, examples, and case studies are for illustrative purposes only; any resemblance to actual persons, living or dead, is purely coincidental. Title: Life After Osteoporosis Diagnosis: How to Rebuild Strength and Confidence at Any Age Author: Elena Forti

Disclaimer

This book is for education and general information only. It is not medical advice, it is not a diagnostic tool, and it is not a substitute for care from a qualified clinician. Reading this book does not create a clinician patient relationship with the author or the publisher. Health information can change quickly and may not apply to your situation. Always speak with your doctor, pharmacist, or licensed health professional about your personal needs before you start, stop, or change any exercise program, medication, supplement, diet, or test schedule.

Exercise and movement carry risk. If you have pain, dizziness, shortness of breath, chest discomfort, sudden weakness, or any symptom that worries you, stop the activity and seek medical attention. If you suspect a fracture or a medical emergency, call your local emergency number at once. People with vertebral fractures, severe osteoporosis, balance problems, or other health conditions need individualized guidance. Ask your clinician or a trained therapist to help you adapt the activities in this book to your abilities and to your environment.

Information about medications, dosages, side effects, interactions, and monitoring is presented for general understanding only. Decisions about prescriptions must be made with your clinician, using your medical history, your current tests, and your preferences. Mentions of specific products or services are examples, not endorsements. Trademarks and brand names belong to their owners.

While every effort was made to ensure accuracy, the author and publisher make no guarantees and accept no responsibility for errors or omissions. By using this book you agree that the author, the publisher, and any contributors are not liable for any loss, injury, or damages that may arise from the use of the information provided. Your choices are your own. Use this book as a starting point for informed conversations with your healthcare team.

Chapter 1

Recognizing Hidden Osteoporosis: You Are Not Your Diagnosis

Osteoporosis is often called a silent condition because it develops slowly and quietly. Many people discover it after a routine scan or a minor incident, not because they felt something break inside. If you have just received a diagnosis, it is normal to feel worried. You may wonder if your daily life must shrink. The short answer is no. You can live normally with osteoporosis when you learn how your bones work, how risk is managed, and what choices make you stronger week by week. Your diagnosis is information, not a sentence.

Let us start with what osteoporosis is in simple words. Bone is living tissue. It is not a dry stick. It has a structure like a sponge covered by a shell. Inside this sponge, tiny beams of bone are constantly renewed. Two types of cells do this work. Osteoclasts remove older bone. Osteoblasts build new bone. This process is called remodeling. In youth the system is in balance. With aging, hormones, genetics, and lifestyle, the scale may tip so that a little more bone is removed than rebuilt. Over time the sponge loses some beams. This can reduce bone density and weaken the structure. Because this change is microscopic, you do not feel it while it happens. This is why osteoporosis can remain hidden until a scan or a fracture reveals it.

Knowing that the process is slow brings an important message. If loss took years, improvement will also take time but it is possible. Many people ask if bone density can increase. For many, yes. The amount of change differs from person to person. Some see modest gains, others see stable numbers with better strength and balance, which is just as important because fractures are not caused by numbers alone. Fracture risk comes from a mix of bone strength, muscle strength, balance, vision, medications, home safety, and how you move. When we improve these factors, life becomes safer and more open.

A common fear is whether sports and play are still allowed. Safe activity is not only allowed, it is essential. Movement signals your bones and muscles to stay strong. Walking, brisk walking, stair climbing, and short bouts of gentle jogging on even ground can be safe for many people. Strength training is a key lever because muscles pull on bone and this mechanical pull is one of the strongest signals for bone formation. If you have never trained, you can start with bodyweight, light dumbbells, or resistance bands. Bands are helpful and can maintain strength. Over time, adding some external load, like dumbbells or a barbell under guidance, can create a stronger signal. The right weight is the weight you can move with steady posture and no sudden pain while keeping a smooth breath. You do not need to chase heavy numbers. You need gradual, repeatable effort.

What about yoga or Pilates. These practices can help flexibility, breathing, and body awareness. They can be safe when you choose versions that respect the spine. Avoid deep forward bends, loaded twists, and fast roll downs, especially if you have low bone density in the spine. Focus on neutral spine, long back, and controlled movements. A trained instructor who understands osteoporosis can show safe variations.

If you love to travel, you can continue to travel. Planning reduces risk. Pack light bags with wheels, choose shoes with grip, ask for aisle seats so you can stand easily, and use handrails without rushing. Take breaks to stand and walk. If you lift a suitcase, keep it close to your body and bend at the hips and knees, not from the waist. These small choices make a big difference and let you enjoy the journey.

Many grandparents ask if they can lift their grandchildren. In most cases, yes, with good technique and appropriate pacing. Bring the child close, plant your feet, exhale as you stand, and avoid twisting with load. If you have a recent vertebral fracture, you need a period of healing guided by your clinician. After the acute phase, gradual strength work helps you return to lifting safely. The timeline is individual. The signal that you are ready is a combination of reduced pain, improved posture control, and a clinician's clearance.

People often want to know what prevents everyday fractures. Home is the best place to start because it is where you spend most time. Good lighting, clear floors, stable rugs, and grab bars in the bathroom cut risk. Outside, choose shoes that do not slip, watch for uneven curbs, and use a backpack instead of a shoulder bag so your hands are free. Equally important is how you move. Keep a long spine when you pick up objects. Hinge at the hips, bend the knees, and keep items close to your center. Avoid quick, rounded stoops with rotation when you are holding a load. These habits protect vertebrae and help you feel in control.

Posture and balance are skills that can improve at any age. Think of posture as tall and relaxed rather than stiff. Imagine a string lifting the crown of your head while your ribs soften down and your pelvis stays neutral. Practice standing near a wall with your heels a small step away. Touch the wall lightly with the back of your head and upper back. Breathe slowly and feel how your weight spreads through both feet. For balance, start with a safe support nearby. Stand on one foot for a few seconds and switch sides. Turn your head gently while you keep your chest tall. These simple drills, done most days, can reduce falls.

What if you do not want medications. It is your right to choose. Some people do very well with a plan based on exercise, protein rich food, calcium and vitamin D, and safer daily habits. Others have a fracture history or very low scores where medications can be useful. The best choice is informed and personal. If you decide to wait, agree with your clinician on a period of structured training and nutrition, then reassess with a new scan. This keeps the decision active and based on evidence.

How much calcium do you need. Most adults need around 1000 to 1200 milligrams per day from food and supplements combined. Aim to cover most of it with food like dairy, fortified plant milks, tofu set with calcium, small fish with bones, leafy greens, and nuts.

Vitamin D helps you absorb calcium. Many adults need a supplement of vitamin D, especially in months with little sun. Magnesium, vitamin K2, and adequate protein also support bone. Collagen can help some people with joint comfort and may contribute amino acids for tissue repair, but it is not a replacement for protein rich meals. Supplements are tools. Use them to fill gaps after you have built a strong base with food.

You may have heard of DEXA and TBS. DEXA measures bone mineral density and gives a T score that compares your bones to those of a healthy younger adult. TBS looks at the texture of the vertebrae on the same images and gives extra insight into bone quality. Results can change between tests because machines are different, your hydration can vary, positioning can differ, and real biological change takes time. Use the same center when you can and test at intervals your clinician suggests so trends are easier to read.

A frequent question is whether walking alone is enough. Walking is a healthy habit for heart, mood, and general fitness. For bones, walking maintains but often does not increase density on its own, especially at the hips and spine. When you add strength training and short, purposeful bursts of higher effort, the signal becomes stronger. Resistance bands are a good start and can be enough for maintenance. To build bone in many adults, some progressive external load is often needed. You can reach this with dumbbells, kettlebells, or gym machines done with careful form.

If you have a vertebral fracture, can you train. Yes, with guidance. Early on, focus on pain control, posture, breathing, and gentle hip and leg strength while you avoid heavy spinal flexion. As healing progresses, load can return in a stepwise way. You begin with isometric holds and light resistance, then progress to moderate loads that you can control without pain. The moment to lift again depends on healing, symptoms, and medical advice. Moving well is part of recovery.

To live normally with osteoporosis, you do not need to become a different person. You add smart habits to the life you already enjoy. You learn to organize your home, to stand tall, to train with intention, to fuel your body well, and to choose the right tools. Confidence grows when you see what you can do. In the next chapters you will learn the details of bone biology, risk, tests, treatments, and training methods. For now, remember this. Your bones are alive. They respond to care. With patience and steady steps, you can reclaim strength and trust in your body.

Chapter 2

Bone Anatomy and the Remodeling Cycle in Plain English

To take confident steps after an osteoporosis diagnosis, it helps to know what your bones are made of and how they renew themselves. Think of bone as a smart material. It is strong like a bridge yet alive like a garden. It holds you up, protects your organs, stores minerals, and houses bone marrow where blood cells begin. This living system changes every day in response to how you move, what you eat, your hormones, and your age.

Let us start with the structure. Each bone has two main parts. The outer shell is called cortical bone. It is dense and smooth and gives bones their hard surface. The inner section is called trabecular bone. It looks like a sponge with a network of tiny beams and plates. Those beams are arranged along the lines of stress. When you stand, walk, or lift, forces travel through the skeleton. The internal beams line up to carry that load. The hip and the spine have a lot of this inner spongy bone, which is why they respond to training but are also more sensitive to loss.

Zoom in further and you find a mix of minerals and protein. Calcium and phosphorus form crystals that make bone rigid. Collagen, a long flexible protein, gives bone a little bend so it does not crack under every impact. Water and other proteins complete the matrix. When collagen and minerals are balanced, bone is both strong and tough, like reinforced concrete with steel bars inside. With osteoporosis there is less mineral per area and fewer internal beams, so the structure becomes thinner and more fragile.

Now to the most important part for your daily life. Bone is never still. It renews itself through a cycle called remodeling. Two groups of cells do the work. Osteoclasts are the cleanup crew. They gently dissolve a small patch of older bone. Osteoblasts are the builders. They fill that patch with fresh bone. A third cell type called the osteocyte sits inside the bone and acts as a sensor. When you move, the fluid inside the bone shifts and the osteocyte senses this. It sends signals that tell the cleanup crew and the builders where to work. This is why movement matters. Without regular mechanical signals, the system becomes quiet and more tissue is removed than rebuilt.

In childhood and young adulthood remodeling builds more bone than it removes. Around midlife, hormonal changes, lower activity, and genetics can shift the balance. In women the drop in estrogen at menopause speeds up the cleanup crew. In men testosterone and other hormones also change with age. If the builders cannot keep up, the internal beams thin or break. You do not feel this as it happens because the changes occur at a microscopic scale. Over time the inner network becomes less connected and the shell may thin too. That is how hidden osteoporosis develops.

The good news is that the cycle remains responsive at any age. When you place safe, progressive load through your body, the osteocytes notice. They send signals to favor building. Bones adapt slowly, like a savings account that grows with steady deposits. You will not see large changes in a few weeks. You can see meaningful change across months and years. What you do most days is what matters.

People often ask which exercises increase bone density. Strength training that loads the hips and spine is the most direct stimulus. Think of movements like squats to a safe chair height, hip hinges where you keep your back long, step ups, and presses for the upper body. You can start with bodyweight and resistance bands to learn positions. Bands can maintain strength and are useful when you travel. To build density for many adults, adding some external weight is helpful because it creates a stronger signal at the bone. The right amount is personal. Choose a weight you can lift with good posture, smooth breathing, and no sharp pain. When a set feels steady and you could do a little more, you can increase the load slightly. This is called progressive overload and it is the language bones understand.

What about walking. Walking is great for your heart, your mood, and your stamina. For bone density, walking maintains more than it builds, especially at the spine. If walking is your favorite activity, keep it, and add short bursts of faster pace on level ground if your joints allow. Combine your walks with two or three short strength sessions each week and you give your bones the message they need.

Are yoga and Pilates safe. They can be when you choose shapes that respect the spine and avoid deep forward bends and loaded twists. Focus on long aligned posture, controlled breathing, and stable hips and shoulders. These practices improve balance and body awareness, which reduces falls. Lower fall risk means lower fracture risk even if your bone density number stays the same for a while.

Can you live normally with osteoporosis while this remodeling is going on. Yes. Once you understand that your bones listen to daily signals, you can shape those signals. Sit tall and change positions often during the day. When you pick something up, hinge from your hips, bend your knees, and keep the object close to your body. When you carry groceries or lift a grandchild, bring the load close, plant your feet, and avoid twisting while lifted. These small rules protect the internal beams of the spine.

People also ask about training after a vertebral fracture. The bone needs time to heal. During the early phase you focus on pain control, breathing, gentle hip and leg strength, and posture practice. As healing progresses and your clinician gives the green light, you return to gradual loading. Start with isometric holds, then light resistance, then moderate weights that you can control without pain. Remodeling will respond to these steps. Recovery is not about perfect numbers. It is about function returning smoothly.

Nutrition plays a direct role because minerals come from your plate. Most adults aim for about 1000 to 1200 milligrams of calcium per day from food and supplements combined. Try to meet most of this with meals. Dairy, fortified plant milks, tofu set with calcium, canned fish with bones, leafy greens, almonds, and sesame paste are common choices. Vitamin D helps you absorb calcium. Many adults benefit from a vitamin D supplement, especially in low sun months. Magnesium supports the mineral matrix and vitamin K2 helps direct calcium toward the skeleton. Adequate protein gives your body the building blocks for collagen and muscle. Collagen supplements may support joint comfort for some people. Use supplements to fill gaps rather than as a replacement for balanced meals.

How do DEXA and TBS connect to what you feel day to day. DEXA measures the amount of mineral in a region and gives you a T score. TBS analyzes the quality of the spongy structure in the spine by reading texture in the same images. Scores can vary between centers and over time for reasons that are not about real change, such as positioning or hydration. Try to test on the same machine when possible and discuss trends with your clinician rather than reacting to a single number. Remember that fractures depend on more than density. Balance, muscle strength, reaction time, vision, home safety, and medication side effects all matter. This is empowering because you can influence many of these factors starting today.

A common concern is whether lifting weights is safe. It is safe when you respect form, progress slowly, and stop if you feel sharp pain, dizziness, or unusual symptoms. Good training feels like steady effort, not strain in the spine. Work with a coach or therapist who understands osteoporosis if you can. If you prefer to train alone, choose simple movements, keep your spine long, and move with control. Two short sessions each week can make a real difference for bone and balance.

Finally, let us tie anatomy and behavior together. The inner beams of your bones are like paths in a garden. If you walk the same safe paths again and again, they stay clear and strong. If you leave them unused, grass grows and the way becomes weak. Every time you stand up tall, every time you do a careful squat, every time you carry a bag close to your body, you tell the osteocytes that these paths matter. They call the builders to lay down new material along those lines. With patience and practice, your skeleton becomes a more reliable partner. You do not need perfection. You need regular, kind signals that add up.

In the next chapter we will look at who is most at risk and why. For now, remember that your bones are listening. The garden grows where you place your steps.

Chapter 3

Who Is at Risk and Why: Family, Hormones, Aging

Understanding risk does not mean living in fear. It means knowing what you can change and what you can plan for. Osteoporosis develops from a mix of biology and daily life. Some pieces you inherit, like eye color. Others depend on how you move, eat, sleep, and manage health conditions. When you see the full picture, you can decide what to do first and you can speak with your clinician in a clear way.

Let us start with family history. If a parent or a close relative had a hip fracture or was told they had osteoporosis, your risk is higher. Genes shape bone size, bone density, and how quickly bone turns over. They also influence height, body shape, and even how your body uses calcium and vitamin D. You cannot change your parents, yet family history is still useful. It tells you to be proactive sooner. If your mother or grandmother had a hip fracture, you can begin strength training, balance practice, and nutrition work now rather than later. You can ask for a baseline DEXA and you can repeat it at intervals that make sense for your age and history. Family history does not decide your future. It simply says pay attention.

Hormones play a central role. In women the drop in estrogen around menopause speeds up bone resorption. The cleanup crew works faster and the builders cannot always keep up. This is why bone density can decline more quickly in the first years after periods stop. In men testosterone and other hormones change with age and can lead to similar patterns, often later in life. Thyroid and parathyroid hormones also affect bone. Too much thyroid hormone, whether from the gland itself or from medication that is slightly too high, can accelerate loss. Parathyroid hormone regulates calcium in the blood. If it is out of balance, bone can be used as a calcium bank too often. Cortisol, the stress hormone, matters as well. Long term high levels, including from steroid medications like prednisone, signal the skeleton to let go of tissue. Understanding hormones helps you see why medical checks are important in a bone health plan.

Aging is another strong factor, but age is not destiny. As we age we often move less and we lose some muscle strength. Muscles protect bone. When muscle falls, balance and reaction time can slow. Falls become more likely and fractures become more common. Aging also changes the inner structure of bone. The tiny beams inside become thinner and less connected. The outer shell can thin. These changes can happen without symptoms. The good news is that bone and muscle still respond to training and to protein rich meals across the lifespan. People in their seventies and eighties get stronger when they train with care. Better strength and balance lower fall risk even before the next scan shows a change.

Certain health conditions raise risk. Celiac disease, inflammatory bowel disease, and other conditions that affect absorption can reduce the nutrients available for bone. Rheumatoid arthritis and other inflammatory conditions increase turnover and often require medications that affect bone. Eating disorders, very low body weight, and long periods of missed periods in younger years leave a lasting mark. Type 1 diabetes and some neurological conditions also increase risk, in part through falls. If any of these apply to you, it is even more important to build a simple daily routine that feeds bone and protects you during movement.

Medications can be part of the story. Glucocorticoids used for asthma, autoimmune disease, or after transplants are well known for their effects on bone when used for long periods. Some treatments for breast or prostate cancer change hormone levels and can reduce bone density. Certain anti seizure drugs and stomach acid medicines may play a role in some people. None of this means you should stop a needed medication on your own. It means you and your clinician can balance benefits and risks and can add protective steps, such as earlier strength training, vitamin D, calcium through food, and fall prevention work at home.

Lifestyle is a powerful lever because it is yours to shape. Tobacco reduces blood flow to bone and interferes with the building process. Heavy alcohol use increases falls and changes how bone cells work. Very low physical activity leaves the osteocytes with few signals to build. Low protein intake makes it harder to maintain muscle and collagen. The path forward is simple and practical. Shift toward smoke free living. Keep alcohol in a light to moderate range if you drink. Move most days. Include two or three short strength sessions each week. Aim for enough protein spread through the day and base your meals on whole foods that include calcium sources.

Body size and shape matter. People with very low body weight have less bone mass to draw on and often lower hormone levels. This does not mean weight gain is always the answer. It means that a healthy weight for your frame and a steady supply of protein and energy support bone. Very rapid weight loss is hard on the skeleton. If you are planning weight loss for other health reasons, keep your bones in mind. Preserve muscle with strength training and protein and talk with your clinician about timing your DEXA so that results are easier to interpret.

Falls are the final common pathway to many fractures. Even with moderate bone density a hard fall can cause a break. This is why balance, vision, and home safety count as much as the number on the scan. Clear floors, secure rugs, good lighting, and stable shoes help daily. Simple drills such as standing on one foot near a support, heel to toe walking, and getting up from a chair without using your hands build control. If you use medications that make you sleepy or lightheaded, ask whether the timing or dose can be adjusted. If your vision prescription is old, update it. These steps are part of risk management and are within reach for most people.

People often ask how risk relates to sports, travel, and family life. If you enjoy a sport that includes impact or quick direction changes, you can often continue with smart adjustments. Choose even surfaces, warm up well, and keep your spine long during lifts. If you travel, plan routes with fewer stairs when you can, use handrails, pack wheels, and take walking breaks. If you lift grandchildren, bring them close to your body, exhale as you stand, and avoid twisting while you hold them. These habits allow joy and safety to live together.

Nutrition touches risk in a direct way. Many adults need about 1000 to 1200 milligrams of calcium per day. It is best to cover most of this with food. Add vitamin D when needed, especially in low sun months. Magnesium and vitamin K2 support the matrix and help direct calcium to the right place. Most people should focus first on protein at each meal and a variety of whole foods. Supplements are tools for gaps rather than the base of the plan.

Screening helps you see where you stand. A DEXA scan gives bone density at the hip and spine. TBS can add information about the quality of the spongy structure in the spine. Results change for many reasons, including positioning and machine differences. Try to use the same center when possible. Discuss trends with your clinician instead of reacting to a single number. If your risk is high because of family history, early menopause, past fractures, or medications that affect bone, ask about earlier or more frequent scanning. Testing is not about fear. It is about guiding your decisions.

What if you do not want medications. That choice is personal and valid. Some people prefer to begin with movement, nutrition, and fall prevention and then review progress. Others have very low scores or a fracture history where medication can lower risk faster. A good plan respects your values and keeps communication open. Set a time frame for action. Train, eat well, create a safer home, and then repeat the scan. Make the next decision with fresh data.

The big picture is simple. Risk comes from family, hormones, aging, health conditions, medications, body size, and daily habits. You hold real power in how you move, how you fuel your body, how you set up your home, and how you ask for care. Small steps done often build protection. You do not have to change everything at once. Choose one action today that makes your bones, your muscles, or your balance stronger. Repeat it tomorrow. Over time these actions shape your risk far more than fear ever could.

Chapter 4

Testing Your Bones: DEXA vs TBS and Why Results Change

When you first see a bone scan report it can look like a puzzle full of letters and numbers. Once you know what each piece means, the picture becomes clear and useful. DEXA and TBS are tools that look at your bones in different ways. DEXA measures how much mineral is packed into a small area. TBS reads the texture of the spongy bone in your spine to estimate quality. They answer related questions. DEXA tells you about bone quantity. TBS adds information about how well the inner network is organized. Used together they guide decisions better than either one alone.

Let us start with DEXA. The scan is painless and quick. It uses a very low dose of X rays to measure bone mineral density in specific regions. The most common sites are the lumbar spine and the hip. Some people are also tested at the forearm when the hip and spine are not suitable or when hyperparathyroidism is a concern. The report shows a T score and sometimes a Z score. The T score compares your density to that of a healthy younger adult. A result of minus 2.5 or lower meets the definition used for osteoporosis. Osteopenia or low bone mass is between minus 1.0 and minus 2.5. The Z score compares you to people your age and sex and is useful when a younger person has low density or when secondary causes are suspected. These numbers are not grades for your worth. They are data points that help you and your clinician choose the next step.

Now TBS. Trabecular Bone Score is not a separate scan. It is software that analyzes the same images from your DEXA of the lumbar spine. The inner part of vertebrae is made of a web of tiny beams. When that web is dense and well connected the texture looks different to the software than when the web is thin and broken. The TBS value reflects that texture. A higher TBS suggests better microarchitecture. A lower TBS suggests more fragile structure. TBS helps explain why two people with the same T score can have different fracture risks. One person may have a stronger inner web and another may not. This extra lens is especially helpful when degenerative changes in the spine make the DEXA value look artificially high because TBS is less affected by those changes.

Which test is more accurate is a common question. It is more helpful to think of them as complementary rather than in competition. DEXA is the standard for diagnosing osteoporosis and for tracking changes in bone mineral density over time. TBS adds context about quality that DEXA alone cannot see. If your DEXA shows low bone mass but your TBS is relatively strong, your plan may focus on strength and balance with careful monitoring. If your DEXA looks borderline yet TBS is low, you and your clinician might lean toward a more active treatment plan because the structure looks fragile even if the quantity is not very low.

Results change from one test to the next for many reasons. Some are about real biological change. Most are about measurement conditions. Positioning matters. If your legs are not supported the same way under the knees, your spine may arch differently and the measured area may shift. If your hips are rotated a little more or less, the region of interest changes and the numbers change with it. Machine type matters because different manufacturers and even different devices from the same company have slightly different calibrations. Hydration and body weight can influence soft tissue thickness and change how X rays pass through, which can nudge values up or down. Spinal arthritis, calcified blood vessels near the spine, scoliosis, and old compression fractures can raise the apparent density of the spine region on DEXA even when the inner web is not strong. Metal near the scan area, belts, buttons, and thick clothing can also create artifacts. All of these factors can make a small difference from test to test and sometimes a difference big enough to look like change when nothing important has happened inside the bone.

Because of these issues professionals use a simple idea called least significant change. Think of it as the size of difference that must be passed before we call it real. Each center calculates this based on how precise their machine and technique are. As a rough picture, small changes within a few percent may sit inside the noise, while larger changes that repeat on the next test are more likely to be real. This is another reason to scan at the same center with the same machine and the same positioning whenever possible. Consistency lets you see a true trend rather than a zigzag of noise.

Here is how to prepare and what to expect, explained in plain steps without a checklist. Wear clothing without metal zippers or buttons and remove belts and jewelry. Bring earlier reports if you have them. Tell the technician if you have had back pain, a known fracture, a hip replacement, or scoliosis. Mention recent tests that used contrast or barium because they can leave traces that confuse the image. Try not to take a large calcium tablet right before the scan because tablets in the stomach can show up as a bright spot. You will lie still while the arm of the scanner passes over you. The team will position your legs on a support to flatten the lower spine and will roll your legs inward for the hip scan so that the correct area is measured. The scan is quick and does not hurt.

Reading the report becomes easier with a few anchors. Look at the sites measured. Check whether your center considers the same vertebrae as last time because sometimes a level is excluded if arthritis or a fracture distorts the reading. Compare T scores at the hip and the spine but give extra weight to the hip if the spine is affected by degenerative change. Look for the precision or least significant change section so you know how much difference counts as real at that center. If TBS is included, read its category alongside the spine T score to form a fuller picture of quality plus quantity. If the report mentions Vertebral Fracture Assessment, it means the team also took side images to look for hidden compression fractures. This can be valuable when height has dropped or when back pain has a new pattern.

People often ask how often to repeat the test. The answer depends on your situation. After starting a new treatment or a structured exercise program, repeating the scan after one to two years can show a trend. If your risk is lower, a longer gap can make sense. Scanning too often invites noise and worry without giving better guidance. Agree on timing with your clinician based on your history, your age, your medications, and whether you have had fractures. Remember that function matters as much as numbers. Stronger legs, better balance, and fewer near falls are wins even before the next scan.

Another common question is whether walking, bands, weights, yoga, or Pilates will move the needle on these tests. They can, over time, when done with enough stimulus and consistency. Walking keeps you active and supports heart health, but it rarely raises spine density by itself. Bands help maintain strength and are useful when traveling. Weights that you lift with good form and slow progression give the strongest signal to bones at the hip and spine. Yoga and Pilates support posture and balance when you avoid deep forward bends and fast roll downs. All of these choices reduce falls and protect the spine, which is equally important because fewer falls mean fewer fractures regardless of the exact number on the page.

If you have had a vertebral fracture, you can still use DEXA and TBS to track your path. Let the team know about the fracture so they can interpret the spine numbers correctly or exclude affected levels. Focus on hip results for trends, and use TBS to understand the quality of the remaining vertebrae. Train gently at first, then more firmly as healing allows, and feed your recovery with protein, calcium rich foods, and vitamin D as needed. Set your goals around function and confidence while the numbers catch up.

In the end, these tests are tools that serve you. They are snapshots, not verdicts. Choose the same center when possible, prepare simply, and read the results in context. Pair DEXA for quantity with TBS for quality. Track trends rather than single points. Use what you learn to fine tune your training, your nutrition, and your daily habits. When you do this, the report becomes a guide that supports a full life rather than a reason to worry.

Chapter 5

Treatment Choices: Medications, Outcomes, and Non Drug Paths

Choosing a treatment path is not a one time decision. It is a conversation that changes as your life changes. The goal is simple. You want fewer fractures and more freedom. There are two broad paths that often work best together. One path uses medications to shift the biology of bone. The other uses daily habits and training to change how forces move through your body and how likely you are to fall. You can start on either path. You can combine them. You can also move between options as your needs evolve.

Let us begin with what medications do in plain words. Some drugs slow the cleanup crew that removes older bone. These are called antiresorptives. When removal slows, the builders can fill in more, and the balance improves. Bisphosphonates are a common family in this group. Examples include alendronate as a weekly pill and zoledronic acid as a yearly infusion. They are often used first because they are well studied and can lower the chance of spine and hip fractures. Another antiresorptive is denosumab, given as a shot every six months. It acts on a signal that tells the cleanup cells to be active. When that signal is blocked, removal slows. These medicines do not make bone overnight. They change the pace of the cycle so that your inner network can stabilize.

Other drugs act more like builders. They are called anabolic agents. Teriparatide and abaloparatide are daily injections that stimulate new bone formation. Romosozumab is a monthly injection that has a dual effect. It increases building and also slows removal for a period of time. Anabolic treatments are often used for people with very low bone density or with recent fractures, especially in the spine, because they can raise density more quickly. After a course of an anabolic drug, people usually move to an antiresorptive to hold the gains.

Hormone therapy can also play a role for some women close to menopause when symptoms are strong and fracture risk is a concern. It can help slow loss but it is not right for everyone. The decision depends on age, personal and family history, and risk factors for heart disease, stroke, and breast cancer. Calcitonin is used less often today because it is less effective for fracture prevention, though it may be used short term for pain relief after an acute vertebral fracture. Your clinician will guide you through these nuances.

People worry about side effects and that is reasonable. Serious effects are rare but they receive a lot of attention. With oral bisphosphonates, stomach upset can happen if the pill is taken without enough water or if you lie down too soon after swallowing it. Taking the tablet first thing with a full glass of water and staying upright for thirty to sixty minutes helps. With infusions you can feel flu like for a day or two. Denosumab can lower blood calcium if vitamin D and calcium intake are low, so those need attention. Very rare events like osteonecrosis of the jaw and atypical femur fractures have been reported with long term antiresorptive use. The absolute risk is low compared to the risk of hip fracture in untreated people at high risk. Dental checks and good oral hygiene help. If you need a major dental procedure, you and your clinician can plan timing.

An important detail with denosumab is that stopping it suddenly can lead to a rebound increase in bone turnover. This can raise fracture risk, especially in the spine. If denosumab is stopped, it should be followed by another antiresorptive to hold the gains. With bisphosphonates, some people can take a break after a few years because the medicine binds to bone and keeps working for a while. This pause is called a drug holiday and depends on your fracture risk and your scan results. Anabolic drugs are used for limited courses and then followed by an antiresorptive to keep the new bone.

What outcomes can you expect. Medications reduce the chance of fractures when used as directed and when paired with adequate calcium, vitamin D, and strength work. Spine density can rise within a year. Hip density changes more slowly. The amount of improvement varies. Some people see several percentage points of gain. Others see stability, which is still a win if you were losing density before. Remember that fewer falls and safer movement can lower fracture risk even if the bone number changes slowly. Track both numbers and function. Ask yourself how often you trip, how steady you feel on one foot, and how confident you are when you lift a suitcase. These are outcomes that matter in daily life.

Can you improve without medications. Many people can improve function and reduce risk with a plan based on training, nutrition, and safer habits. The key is structure and consistency. If you choose a non drug path, set a clear timeline with your clinician. Train two or three times per week with a focus on legs, hips, and back. Aim for good form and gradual progression. Add brisk walking or short power intervals if your joints allow. Eat protein at each meal and reach the calcium range your clinician recommends. Check vitamin D and supplement if levels are low. Make your home safer with better lighting, clear floors, and secure rugs. After an agreed period, often one to two years, repeat your scan and review your progress together. This approach respects your choice while keeping the plan evidence based.

How much can bone density improve without medications. Gains are usually modest and depend on where you start, your training stimulus, your nutrition, and your hormones. Some people see small increases at the hip and spine with consistent strength work. Others hold steady and build muscle and balance, which still lowers the chance of a fall and a fracture. Think of bone as one piece of a bigger system. Stronger muscles protect joints and absorb forces. Better posture spreads load across the spine. Quicker reactions prevent stumbles from becoming falls.

Where do supplements fit. Start with food first. Most adults need about 1000 to 1200 milligrams of calcium per day from diet and supplements combined. If food falls short, a simple calcium supplement can fill the gap. Vitamin D helps you absorb calcium. Many adults benefit from a vitamin D supplement, especially in months with little sun. Magnesium supports the mineral matrix and vitamin K2 helps guide calcium into bone tissue. Collagen can support joint comfort and provides amino acids that your body can use, but it does not replace a protein rich meal. If you take medications, review possible interactions with your clinician or pharmacist. Supplements are additions. They do not replace training, food quality, or medical care when needed.

Are weights safe. They are safe when you respect technique and progress in small steps. Keep your spine long, hinge from the hips when you bow forward, and avoid deep rounded bends with load. Choose a weight that feels challenging by the end of a set while you can still control the movement and breathe steadily. Bands are helpful when you start or when you travel. They maintain strength and can be part of a full plan. To change bone density for many adults, some external load is usually needed. Machines at the gym can be a friendly way to add weight with control. Walking is healthy for many reasons and should stay in your week, yet it rarely raises spine density by itself.

Combine walking with strength work for the best signal.

If you have had a vertebral fracture, medications may be especially helpful early on to stabilize the biology while you rebuild strength. Training will still be part of your recovery. During the first phase focus on posture, breathing, and gentle hip and leg work. When pain settles and your clinician clears you, add controlled loading. Avoid quick roll downs and heavy twists. Use your breath as a guide. Exhale during effort and keep movements smooth.

How do you decide among all these paths. Start with your values and your risk. Ask yourself how you feel about medicines, how likely you are to follow a program at home, and what matters most in your daily life. Bring your scan results, your fracture history, and your questions to your appointment. A good plan is one that you can follow. If you begin with non drug steps, set checkpoints. If you begin with medication, support it with training, food, and fall prevention so the benefits are larger. Review your plan each year or after any major change such as a new fracture or a new medication for another condition.

The message is hopeful. You have more than one way to protect your bones. Medications can lower fracture risk when used wisely. Training and daily habits make you stronger and steadier. Nutrition gives your body what it needs to rebuild. Together these choices create a path where you can live fully, travel, play with family, and move with confidence while your bones adapt over time.

Chapter 6

Food for Strong Bones: How Much Calcium You Need and Best Foods

Food is one of the most encouraging parts of bone health because you make choices several times a day. Each meal is a chance to support your skeleton and your muscles. You do not need a perfect diet. You need steady habits that are easy to repeat. This chapter explains how much calcium most people need, where to find it in everyday food, and how vitamin D, K2, magnesium, protein, and collagen fit into the picture. You will see that a simple plate can be powerful.

Let us begin with calcium. Most adults aim for about 1000 to 1200 milligrams per day from food and supplements combined. The exact target depends on age, sex, and medical advice. Think of this as a daily range rather than a strict number. Your bones do not know what day of the week it is. They care about your average over time. Try to meet most of your calcium needs from food and use supplements only to fill gaps.

Which foods help the most. Dairy foods are a straightforward source for many people. Milk, yogurt, and hard cheeses provide calcium in a form your body absorbs well. If you choose plant milks, look for ones that are fortified with calcium and vitamin D and shake the carton before pouring so the added minerals do not settle. Tofu can be a strong source when it is set with calcium salts. Check the label for calcium sulfate or calcium chloride. Small fish eaten with the bones such as sardines and canned salmon add both calcium and protein. Leafy greens like kale and bok choy offer calcium with good absorption. Spinach is nutritious but its calcium is less available because of oxalates, so enjoy spinach for its other benefits and choose different greens for calcium. Almonds, sesame paste, and chia add smaller amounts that contribute over the week.

Protein matters as much as calcium because bone is not made of minerals alone. It has a protein framework of collagen that minerals attach to. Aim to include protein at each meal. Eggs, fish, poultry, lean meats, dairy, tofu, tempeh, beans, lentils, and edamame are all helpful. A steady supply of protein supports muscle repair after training and helps you maintain strength. Strong muscles protect your bones by absorbing part of the forces of daily life and by improving balance.

Vitamin D is the partner that helps you absorb calcium from the gut. Sunlight on the skin can produce vitamin

D but many adults do not make enough, especially in winter or if they use sunscreen regularly. Foods such as fortified milk, fortified plant milks, and fatty fish contribute some vitamin D but often not enough to meet needs. This is why many people take a simple vitamin D supplement after checking their level with a clinician. Vitamin D supports bone mineralization and also supports muscle function, which lowers fall risk.

Magnesium is a quiet helper in bone health. It is part of the mineral matrix and plays a role in how vitamin D works. You can find magnesium in nuts, seeds, whole grains, beans, and leafy greens. When your meals include these foods most days you likely cover a good part of your needs. If you have cramps, low appetite, or certain medications that affect magnesium, your clinician may suggest a supplement. Food first remains a wise rule.

Vitamin K2 helps guide calcium into bone tissue and away from soft tissues. Fermented foods such as natto are high in K2, and smaller amounts are found in some cheeses. Many people get enough vitamin K from a varied diet, though exact intake varies by food culture. If you are on a blood thinner that interacts with vitamin

K, do not change your intake without medical advice. Consistency is key when managing those medications.

Where does collagen fit. Collagen supplements provide amino acids that your body can use to build connective tissue. Some people notice better joint comfort when they take collagen regularly. Collagen is not a replacement for a protein rich meal, yet it can be a helpful addition, especially for older adults who find it hard to meet protein goals. If you use it, place it alongside meals rather than counting it as your main protein source.

People often ask how to build a simple day of eating that covers bone basics without counting every gram. Start by anchoring each meal around a protein source. Add a calcium rich food. Include a colorful fruit or vegetable. Add a whole grain or another source of energy if your day is active. Breakfast could be yogurt with fruit and a sprinkle of nuts, or fortified soy milk with oats and chia, or eggs with sautéed greens and a piece of whole grain toast. Lunch might be a tofu and vegetable stir fry set with calcium rich tofu, or canned salmon on whole grain crackers with a salad, or a lentil soup with a side of kale. Dinner could be baked sardines with roasted vegetables, chicken with broccoli and brown rice, or a chickpea stew with tahini stirred in. These are not strict menus. They are ideas you can shape to your taste.

Hydration supports overall health and may help with balance and energy. Aim to drink water regularly through the day. Tea and coffee can be part of a healthy pattern when you do not overdo caffeine. If you enjoy alcohol, keep it in a light to moderate range and include food when you drink. Heavy alcohol use increases fall risk and interferes with bone building.

Calcium supplements are common and can be helpful when food does not reach the target. Choose a simple product that provides calcium in a form you tolerate, such as calcium carbonate taken with meals or calcium citrate which is absorbed well even when stomach acid is lower. Split doses across the day if you need more than 500 milligrams from supplements so that absorption is smoother. More is not better. Very high doses are not needed and can cause constipation in some people. Take only what fills the gap between your meals and your daily goal.

How does food connect to the questions you ask about training and daily life. Strong bones and strong muscles come from both movement and nutrition. If you are adding weights or resistance bands, protein becomes even more important. A serving at breakfast, lunch, and dinner helps your muscles rebuild after sessions. If you walk a lot, remember that walking is healthy for your heart but rarely raises spine density by itself. Food choices do not change that, yet they do support the muscle and bone response to your strength training. If you practice yoga or Pilates, good nutrition supports the tissues that hold you in alignment. If you are recovering from a vertebral fracture, enough protein, calcium, and vitamin D can support healing while your training restarts in small steps.

Travel and family life fit into this plan. On the road you can pack calcium rich snacks such as almonds, small cans of fish, or shelf stable fortified plant milks. In restaurants you can add yogurt, leafy sides, or tofu dishes. When you lift grandchildren or suitcases, fuel matters. A well fed body is more resilient and less prone to fatigue. Less fatigue means better form and fewer risky movements.

People sometimes worry that food choices must be perfect to help bone density. That is not true. Patterns matter more than single days. If your week includes many small deposits of calcium and protein and if you keep vitamin D, magnesium, and K2 in mind, you are doing meaningful work. Combine this with your training and your safer home habits and you build a system that protects you from several angles. Your next scan will show part of the story. Your daily confidence will show the rest.

If you are not sure where to start, begin with one change that feels easy. Add a calcium rich food to the meal you eat most often. Check whether your plant milk is fortified. Place a source of protein on every plate. Ask your clinician to check vitamin D if it has been a while. Small steps, repeated, become strong bones over time.

In the next chapter we will look at supplements in more detail so you can decide what to use, what to skip, and how to combine them safely with your medications and your training.

Chapter 7

Supplements Made Simple: D3, K2, Magnesium, Collagen

Supplements can feel confusing. Shelves are full of bottles that promise strong bones and pain free joints. The truth is calmer and more practical. Supplements are tools that fill gaps left by food and sunlight. They support a plan that already includes training, protein, and calcium rich meals. They do not replace those habits. In this chapter you will learn what vitamin D3, vitamin K2, magnesium, and collagen actually do, how to think about dosage with your clinician, how to spot quality, and when to use each product. You will also see how supplements relate to your everyday questions about walking, weights, bands, yoga, travel, and life after a fracture.

Let us start with vitamin D3. Vitamin D helps you absorb calcium from the gut and helps your muscles work well. Many adults have low levels, especially in winter or if they spend little time in direct sun. Food helps but often does not cover the need. Fortified milk and plant milks contribute. Fatty fish helps. Still, a simple D3 supplement is common. The right dose depends on your blood level, your skin, your latitude, your body weight, and your medications. Your clinician can check a 25 hydroxy vitamin D level and suggest a dose to reach and maintain a healthy range. After a few months you can recheck to make sure you are on track. Taking vitamin D with a meal that includes some fat improves absorption. If a weekly or monthly dose is easier for you, ask about that schedule. The goal is steady levels, not quick swings.

Vitamin K2 comes next. K2 helps guide calcium into the skeleton and keeps it away from soft tissues. Your body uses K2 to activate proteins that work like traffic signals for calcium. Fermented foods provide some K2 and certain cheeses contain smaller amounts. Intake varies a lot between people, which is why K2 often appears in bone health blends. If you take a blood thinner that interacts with vitamin K, do not change your intake without medical guidance. Consistency is the key in that situation. For most people who do not take those medicines, a modest K2 supplement alongside D3 can be a reasonable choice. Think of K2 as a helper rather than a lead actor. It works best in the context of adequate D3, calcium from food, and regular training.

Magnesium is a quiet partner that helps more than three hundred reactions in the body. For bones it supports the mineral matrix and influences vitamin D metabolism. Many adults do not reach the recommended intake from food every day. Nuts, seeds, beans, whole grains, and leafy greens provide magnesium, yet routines can drift. A supplement can help when cramps, constipation, low appetite, or certain medications point to low magnesium. Forms like magnesium citrate and magnesium glycinate are often well tolerated. The right amount depends on your diet, your kidneys, and your symptoms. Too much can loosen your bowels. Start low, take it with food, and adjust with your clinician. If you have kidney disease you need medical guidance before using magnesium.

Collagen is different from vitamins and minerals. It is a source of amino acids, mainly glycine, proline, and hydroxyproline. Your body uses these to build connective tissues such as tendons, ligaments, and the protein framework of bone. People often notice that their joints feel more comfortable after several weeks of regular collagen use. Some mix it into coffee or smoothies. Others prefer ready to drink forms. Collagen is not a complete protein. It does not replace the protein from eggs, fish, poultry, dairy, tofu, beans, or lentils. It can be a helpful addition, especially for older adults who find it hard to meet protein targets or for those recovering from a fracture who want extra building blocks. If you use collagen, place it near your training session or a meal so that your body has a steady supply of amino acids when tissues are adapting.

How do you choose products in a crowded market. Focus on simplicity and clarity. Pick single nutrient products when you can so you know what you are taking. Read labels for the exact form and amount. Look for products that are third party tested for purity. Avoid blends that claim to replace exercise or to regrow bone fast. Those promises are not realistic. Your bones respond to daily signals. Supplements support those signals. If you prefer a combined product to reduce the number of pills, choose one that lists D3, K2, and magnesium in sensible amounts rather than megadoses. Keep calcium mostly on your plate, then add a simple tablet to close any gap.

People ask whether supplements can increase bone density by themselves. The answer is that they rarely move the DEXA number without the support of training and adequate protein. Supplements can correct a deficiency that would otherwise block progress. For example, low vitamin D can limit calcium absorption and make strength work less effective. Low magnesium can affect muscle function and sleep. Correcting these gaps can make your plan work better. The DEXA and TBS chapters explain why numbers change and how long real biological change takes. Use that timeline to set realistic expectations.

What about interactions with medications. This is a smart question to bring to your clinician or pharmacist. Calcium can interfere with the absorption of certain thyroid medicines and some antibiotics if taken at the same time. Space them apart when needed. Vitamin D and K2 can interact with some drugs. Magnesium can interact with diuretics and heart medicines. Collagen rarely interacts but powders may contain sweeteners or flavorings that you may wish to avoid. Keep a simple list of what you take and share it during appointments. Update the list when you add or stop a product so that your team can help you avoid conflicts.

How do supplements fit into your daily routine. Tie them to habits you already have. Take D3 with your main meal. Place magnesium with dinner if it helps you sleep, or earlier if you prefer. If you use K2, take it alongside D3. If you use calcium, split the dose so that you do not take more than about five hundred milligrams at once. Combine collagen with a snack after training or stir it into breakfast. Travel with small labeled containers so you keep your routine on the road. If time zones and meals shift, do not worry. Aim for consistency over a week, not perfection each day.

Let us connect supplements to the activities you care about. If you walk daily, D3 and magnesium support muscle function and energy. If you train with weights or bands, protein at each meal and a collagen addition can help your tissues adapt. If you enjoy yoga or Pilates, magnesium may ease cramps and support relaxation, while D3 supports muscle control. If you lift grandchildren or luggage, a well nourished body recovers faster and keeps form under load. If you are healing from a vertebral fracture, adequate D3, calcium from food, and protein support bone repair while your training restarts gently. Supplements do not replace careful movement, but they make the path smoother.

What if you prefer not to take any supplements. You can still make meaningful progress with food and training. Check whether your plant milks are fortified. Use tofu set with calcium. Include small fish with bones. Place protein on every plate. Get outside when safe sunlight is available and your skin allows. Ask your clinician to test vitamin D if you are unsure. If your levels are low, a short course of D3 may be a simple addition that unlocks other gains. The choice remains yours.

Finally, remember that more is not better. The body likes steady, moderate inputs. Megadoses raise the risk of side effects without extra benefit. Keep your plan simple. Eat balanced meals. Move most days. Train with good form. Sleep well. Add D3, K2, magnesium, or collagen when they fit your needs and your tests. Review your choices once or twice a year with your healthcare team. This approach turns a crowded supplement aisle into a small set of helpful tools that support your larger goal. Fewer fractures, more strength, and a life lived with confidence.

Chapter 8

Everyday Safety: How to Avoid Common Fractures at Home and Outside

Staying safe day to day is not about living smaller. It is about choosing how you move and how you set up your world so that strong moments happen more often and risky moments fade. Most fractures come from simple events that can be shaped. A missed step on a dim stair. A twist while lifting a bag. A quick reach from a rounded back. When you change the conditions and your habits, you cut risk without giving up the life you enjoy.

Start with the place where you spend the most time. Home can be a safety net when you set it up with purpose. Light is a powerful protector. Keep rooms bright and switch bulbs that are too dim. Place a small lamp within easy reach of the bed so that night trips are not done in the dark. Clear the paths you walk every day. Shoes by the door can live in a box. Cords can run along walls. Rugs can be secured with non slip backing or removed if they slide. In the bathroom, a simple grab bar near the shower or tub helps you move with confidence. A rubber mat on the floor of the tub or shower reduces slips. If your home has stairs, choose a clear color contrast for the first and last step so your eyes read the change in height quickly.

Your body is part of the setup. Shoes that grip make a difference. Choose soles that feel stable on wet sidewalks and smooth floors. Keep a pair reserved for home if your floors are slippery. Vision is another piece. If your glasses prescription is old, update it so that depth and edges are sharp. If you have bifocals, be careful on stairs because the lower lens can blur your view of the step. Turn your head slightly and look through the top of the lens when you go down. These small adjustments show up as fewer stumbles.

Posture during daily tasks protects the spine. Imagine length from the crown of your head to your tailbone. Let your chest widen without lifting the ribs. Let your lower belly gently support. When you pick something up, move from your hips and knees rather than the waist. Bring the object close to your body before you stand. Exhale as you rise. Avoid twisting while you are holding a load. If you must turn, step your feet to face the new direction, then set the object down. These habits look simple but they keep the internal beams of your vertebrae under friendly forces.

Many people ask if it is safe to lift grandchildren, grocery bags, or laundry baskets. The answer is yes when you plan the lift. Make the load smaller if you can. Use both hands. Stand with your feet at hip width and plant them before you move. Keep the object close to your belly. Breathe out as you stand. If you feel the urge to twist, pause and pivot your feet instead. When you place the object down, keep your spine long and bend your hips and knees. If you are recovering from a vertebral fracture, ask for help during the early healing phase. Return to lifting gradually after your clinician clears you and your training has rebuilt a base.

Kitchens and living rooms are frequent sites of awkward movements. Think through the tasks you do most often and keep heavy items at waist height. Pots and pans can live on the counter or in a drawer that does not require deep bending. Use a reacher tool for low shelves rather than rounding your upper back. When you empty the dishwasher, pull out the racks and step close so that you do not reach from far away. When you make the bed, walk around rather than leaning across. It takes a few extra steps and returns a lot of safety.

Outside the home, sidewalks, steps, and curbs give many people trouble. Look a few steps ahead rather than at your feet. This helps your body plan and keeps your spine in a safer position. If you walk in winter, consider small traction cleats that slip over shoes when the ground is icy. Choose predictable surfaces for brisk walks or intervals. If you enjoy trails, start with smooth paths and build foot strength over time. When you carry bags, split the load between both hands or use a backpack so that your hands are free for railings.

Public transport and travel can stay in your life with simple adjustments. When a bus or train arrives, wait for it to stop before stepping on. Use the handrail and take a solid first step. Keep your bag on your shoulder or your back so that your hands are free. In airports choose a suitcase with wheels and a stable handle. When you lift it into a car trunk, bring it close to your body and use your legs. If the bag is heavy, lift one end onto the edge of the trunk first, then pivot and slide, rather than swinging it from a distance. On planes ask for an aisle seat if standing is easier. Place your bag in the overhead by resting it on the seat back first, then lifting with both hands and a long spine.

Bathrooms, pools, and gyms deserve extra attention because water changes friction. Dry your hands before you reach for a door handle so your grip does not slip. Step onto towels or mats when your feet are wet. At the gym, choose machines and benches that let you keep a long spine. Avoid quick roll downs and deep forward bends with weight. If you are new to strength training, ask for a short tour of the equipment so that set up feels natural and safe. If you use resistance bands, check for small tears before you pull so they do not snap.

Falls often happen during transitions rather than during steady walking. Getting out of bed, rising from a low chair, and turning quickly in a narrow hallway are classic moments. Practice these transitions when you are calm so that the patterns become automatic. Place both feet on the floor before you stand. Lean forward slightly with a long back, push through your feet, and exhale as you rise. When you turn in a small space, take two or three small steps rather than twisting on one foot. If you feel unsteady, touch a wall or countertop lightly with your fingers as you move. These gentle contacts give your balance system extra information.

What about sports and hobbies. They can stay in your life with a few rules. Warm up with slow controlled movements that wake up your hips and shoulders.

Keep your spine long during any lift. Land softly if your activity has small jumps. Avoid quick deep forward bends and rapid twisting under load. If you play tennis or pickleball, work on footwork and spacing so that you reach with your legs rather than rounding your back. If you garden, use a small bench or pad and change positions often. Bring the soil or pot up to a table rather than lifting heavy bags from the ground when possible.

Vision and attention are quiet guardians of safety. When you step into a new space, pause for a breath and scan the floor. Notice wet patches, cords, or uneven edges. Slow down for the first few steps until your body reads the terrain. In crowded places like markets or stations, adopt a steady pace and keep your eyes level so that you see changes early. If you use a phone for music or navigation, stop to look at it. Walking and scrolling together reduce awareness.

People often ask if a cane or walking pole reduces risk or signals weakness. A well fitted cane or a pair of light poles can add stability outdoors, especially on uneven ground. The tool is not a step back. It is a choice that keeps you out in the world. If you are unsure about size and technique, a physical therapist can teach you quickly. The goal is to move with confidence, not to prove anything to anyone.

Nutrition and hydration tie into safety more than most people realize. A steady supply of protein helps you keep muscle that catches you when you trip. Calcium and vitamin D support bone that tolerates small bumps. Water keeps your blood pressure steady when you stand and reduces dizziness. Eat a meal or a snack before long errands so that fatigue does not push you into rushed movements.

Finally, bring curiosity to your own patterns. Notice when and where you feel most steady. Notice which tasks leave your back rounded or your hands full. Adjust one thing at a time. Move a lamp. Shift a rug. Store heavy pots higher. Practice a careful squat near a countertop. Carry smaller bags. Over a few weeks your home and your habits will look different. Fewer stumbles. Fewer awkward lifts. More time spent on the parts of life you love. Safety is not a cage. It is the structure that lets freedom grow.

Chapter 9

Posture and Balance: Spine Protection You Can Trust

Posture and balance are skills, not traits you either have or lack. They change with practice just like strength or flexibility. When you improve these skills you protect the spine, reduce falls, and move with less fear. You do not need special gear or long workouts to begin. You need a clear picture of what safe alignment looks like and short moments of practice woven into your day.

Think of posture as tall and relaxed rather than stiff. Imagine a line that starts at the crown of your head and reaches down through your ears, shoulders, hips, knees, and ankles. That line will not be perfect and it does not have to be. It is a guide that helps your body share load across many tissues so that no single spot carries too much. When you sit, let your weight land on the bones at the base of your pelvis. Slide your rib cage so it floats over your hips and let your shoulders rest wide. When you stand, press the floor gently with all parts of your feet. Feel contact under the heel, the base of the big toe, and the base of the little toe. Let your knees be soft and your head float tall. Small adjustments like these change the forces that travel through the vertebrae.

Breathing connects to posture in a way many people miss. When you breathe only into the top of your chest your ribs lift and your back may arch. When you let the breath expand gently into your sides and back, the ribs move like a quiet umbrella and your spine finds length without strain. Place your hands around your lower ribs and feel them widen on the inhale and return on the exhale. Use this breath to support movements that matter in daily life. Exhale as you stand from a chair, as you lift a bag, or as you step up a curb. Your abdominal wall brings gentle support and your spine stays long.

Protecting your spine during bends and lifts is a skill you can learn at any age. The key idea is to hinge from the hips rather than folding from the waist. When you reach toward the floor, send your hips back as if you are closing a drawer with your seat. Keep your chest open and your back long. Bend your knees enough to keep comfort. Bring the object close before you stand. Push the floor and exhale as you rise. Avoid twisting while you hold weight. If you need to turn, move your feet and whole body together, then place the object down. This pattern keeps the tiny beams inside the vertebrae under friendly compression instead of risky bending and twisting combined.

Balance depends on three systems that talk to each other. Your eyes tell you where you are in space. Sensors in your inner ear track head movement. Nerves in your muscles and joints report pressure and stretch from the ground up. When these systems have clear information they keep you steady without effort. You can train all three. Make your environment easier to read by improving light and reducing clutter. Train your body to feel the ground by spending time in stable shoes and by practicing slow controlled steps. Give your inner ear practice by gently turning your head while you stand tall. Small daily doses teach your nervous system to react faster when life gets unpredictable.

A simple place to start is standing near a wall or countertop so a support is close. Place your feet hip width and find your tall relaxed posture. Let your eyes look level, not at the floor. Breathe slowly. Shift your weight a little forward and back without lifting your heels or toes. Notice how your ankles move. Then shift left and right. After a short time try standing on one foot for a few seconds. Keep a fingertip on the counter if needed. Switch sides and repeat. If this feels easy, turn your head slightly left and right while you balance. If it feels hard, celebrate the training effect and keep the support close. You are teaching your body to stay calm and organized.

Walking can also become balance practice. Think of your foot as a tripod. Land softly on the heel, roll through the arch, and push off the big toe. Let your arms swing gently from the shoulders. Keep your gaze on the horizon so your spine stays long. If sidewalks are uneven, slow down for the first few minutes to read the surface. If you enjoy brisk walking, find a flat route and build pace in short segments. Brisk segments wake up the muscles that stabilize the hips and pelvis, which in turn steadies the spine.

Many people ask about yoga and Pilates when posture and balance feel uncertain. Both practices can help when you choose shapes that respect the spine. Focus on movements that lengthen rather than compress. Choose poses that keep a neutral back, such as a standing forward lean with hands on a countertop where your spine stays long. Avoid deep spinal flexion and quick roll downs, especially if you have low bone density in the spine or a past vertebral fracture. In Pilates look for a teacher who understands how to keep the rib cage heavy and the back long during core work. In yoga choose gentle twists done without rounding and hold shapes with smooth breathing. The goal is control and awareness, not extreme range.

If you have had a vertebral fracture, posture and balance work begin early in recovery. During the first weeks the priority is comfort and calm movement. Practice breathing that expands the ribs without forcing. Lie on your side or back with pillows that let you feel supported. Roll in and out of bed with your spine long by turning as one piece. When you stand, keep the tall relaxed line and take short walks that you can tolerate. As healing progresses, add gentle hip hinges to a chair, short sit to stands, and supported step ups. These actions teach your spine to share load while your confidence returns. Your clinician can guide timing so that you feel safe.

Weights and resistance bands belong in a chapter on posture and balance because strength is the engine that makes alignment easier. When the muscles around your hips, back, and legs are strong, you maintain posture without effort and you correct small slips before they become falls. Start with loads you can control while keeping your neck long and your ribs quiet. If you feel strain in the low back, pause, reset your posture, and reduce the load. Bands are excellent for learning patterns such as a hip hinge or a row. Free weights and machines can add challenge later. The right amount is a weight that feels steady by the end of a set while you can still breathe and talk. Over time increase a little so your body keeps adapting.

Daily life offers many chances to practice without setting aside extra time. When you brush your teeth, stand tall and shift your weight slightly toward one foot, then the other. When you wait for the kettle, place one foot on a small step and feel how that position lengthens your back. When you pick up laundry, hinge at the hips and keep the basket close. When you carry groceries, hold the bags near your body and walk with a quiet breath. These moments rehearse the patterns that protect you when you are tired or distracted.

Attention plays a quiet role. Most stumbles happen when the mind is ahead of the body. Bring your focus to the step you are taking rather than the room you are rushing toward. Pause at doorways and feel your feet. Notice what the floor looks like and whether your shoes grip. If you use a phone for directions, stop to check it rather than looking down while you walk.

Simple awareness supports balance as much as exercises do.

Travel and public spaces add moving parts but the same principles apply. Take a breath before you step off a curb. Keep your head level and your spine long as you rise from airplane seats. Use handrails without apology. Place wheeled suitcases in front of you so your arms are free to guide your steps. When you wake up in a hotel room, stand still for a moment and scan the floor so unfamiliar layouts do not surprise you in the dark. These habits turn new places into safe places.

Confidence grows when practice turns into results you can feel. Notice small wins. Fewer bumps into door frames. Easier turns in the kitchen. A taller feeling when you walk. These are signs that your spine is better protected and your balance system is responding. Pair this work with the nutrition and training chapters you have read. Protein and calcium rich meals fuel the muscles that hold you tall. Vitamin D supports muscle control. Strength workouts teach your body to handle load. All of these pieces talk to each other. Together they reduce fracture risk whether or not the next scan has changed yet.

Posture and balance are not about perfection. They are about friendly alignment and steady practice that fits into real life. You are building a reliable pattern your body can use under stress, when the bus lurches, when a child runs into your arms, when a bag shifts in your hand. With a long spine, calm breath, steady feet, and eyes that look ahead, your body learns to protect you without drama. That is the kind of protection you can trust.

Chapter 10

Training that Builds Bone: Principles, Progression, and Realistic Gains

Bones listen to the language of load. When muscles pull and ground forces travel through your skeleton, tiny sensors inside bone feel the pressure and send signals to rebuild. Training that builds bone is not about punishment or record weights. It is about clear, repeatable messages delivered with good form and patient progression. In this chapter you will learn the principles that matter, how to begin and move forward, how to read your own response, and what results are realistic.

The first principle is specificity. Bones adapt where forces act. If you want to protect your hips and spine, you need movements that load the hips and spine. Simple patterns do this well. Sitting down and standing up from a safe chair. Hinging from the hips while keeping your back long. Stepping up to a stable platform. Pressing weight away from your body with your arms while your ribs stay quiet. These actions spread load through the pelvis, femur, and vertebrae in a way your skeleton understands.

The second principle is progressive overload. Your body changes when you ask a little more than it is used to and then allow time to recover. A little more can mean one extra repetition, a slightly heavier dumbbell, or a slower and more controlled tempo. You do not need large jumps. Small increases that you maintain are safer and build confidence. If a set feels steady and you could do a little more, you are ready to nudge the challenge up next time. If form slips or breath becomes strained, hold the load where it is until it feels smooth again.

The third principle is frequency. Bones like regular signals. Two or three short sessions each week create a rhythm that the remodeling cycle can follow. Sessions can be thirty to forty minutes when you are learning and can be shorter when you are maintaining. Consistency matters more than marathon workouts. When life is busy, a few focused movements are better than skipping the week.

The fourth principle is technique. A long spine protects the tiny beams inside your vertebrae. Keep your head tall, your chest open, and your ribs stacked over your pelvis. When you hinge, send your hips back and bend your knees enough to feel comfortable. Keep the load close to your body. Exhale during effort. Avoid deep forward bends with load and quick twisting while holding weight. This keeps forces friendly and makes training feel safe rather than risky.

How do you start if you are new or returning after a long pause. Begin with bodyweight and light implements to learn the shapes. Practice sit to stands from a chair that lets you succeed. Practice hip hinges with a dowel along your back so you feel length from head to tail. Add step ups at a height that feels easy and stable. Add rows with a band where your shoulder blades glide toward your spine as you pull and relax as you return. When these feel smooth, add a small external load. Dumbbells are simple. Kettlebells work well for hinges and carries. Machines at the gym guide your path and can feel reassuring.

People often ask which exercises increase bone density and by how much. The movements that load the hips and spine are the strongest signal. Squats to a safe chair height. Hip hinges such as a deadlift pattern with a kettlebell held close. Step ups that are steady and controlled. Presses that work the upper body while your trunk stays quiet. Over time these patterns can help raise or stabilize bone density, especially at the hip. The amount of change differs from person to person and grows slowly. Think in months and years, not in weeks. Even when the DEXA number changes modestly, strength, balance, and confidence change faster. Fewer near falls and easier daily lifts are real wins that lower fracture risk.

What about walking. Walking is good for your heart, mood, and general stamina. For bones, walking maintains more than it builds, especially at the spine. Keep walking for health and pair it with strength sessions to send a clearer message to bone. Short brisk segments on level ground can add a power signal if your joints allow, but they do not replace loading for the spine and hips.

Are resistance bands enough. Bands are excellent for learning positions, for travel, and for maintaining strength. They can help you move better and feel steadier. For many adults they are not enough to increase bone density at the hip and spine on their own. You can combine bands with external load so that your body learns control and then receives a stronger mechanical signal.

Are weights safe and how much weight is right. Weights are safe when form is clear and progression is patient. Choose a load that feels challenging near the end of a set while you can still keep your spine long and your breath smooth. For many people this feels like the last two repetitions require focus but do not break form. If you feel pressure in the low back or your shoulders creep toward your ears, pause and adjust. Increase the load only when sets feel steady two sessions in a row. Safety comes from attention to details, not from avoiding weight forever.

Can you train if you have a history of a vertebral fracture. Yes, with timing and guidance. Early on you focus on comfort, posture, and gentle leg strength. As pain settles and your clinician clears you, add isometric holds that build endurance without motion. Then add light resistance with careful hip hinges and step ups. Later you introduce moderate loads that you can control without pain. The moment to lift more is when your posture stays long through the whole set and the next day feels normal. Training is part of recovery and teaches your body that movement is safe again.

Where do yoga and Pilates fit. They support alignment, breathing, and control. Choose versions that avoid deep forward bends, rapid roll downs, and loaded twists. Focus on long lines, stable hips and shoulders, and smooth breath. These practices help posture and balance, which reduce falls. Fewer falls mean fewer fractures even before the next scan changes.

What should older adults or beginners expect in terms of progression. Expect your first gains to be about coordination. Movements feel less awkward. You trust the shapes. Then you notice daily tasks become easier. Rising from a chair. Lifting a small suitcase. Carrying groceries. After several months you may see numbers change on the floor or on a machine. Repetitions increase. Loads inch up. DEXA changes take longer. Stable numbers after years of decline are a real success. Small increases are possible, especially at the hip. The spine can respond too, though it is sensitive to positioning on scans. Track function and confidence alongside the numbers so you see the whole picture.

How do you fit training into a week without turning life upside down. Choose two days that feel natural. Place sessions after a light meal so energy is steady. Warm up with controlled breathing and easy ranges. Train your lower body, your upper body, and your posture. End with a few minutes of balance practice. Walk on the other days and keep a simple routine of home safety and spine friendly habits. If you miss a session, do not double the next one. Return to your normal pattern. The power of training comes from what you repeat, not from intensity spikes.

Travel and family life do not stop your plan. Pack a light band and use hotel chairs for sit to stands and hinges. Choose a room with a small gym if possible and use machines to keep patterns alive. When you lift grandchildren, treat the moment like training. Bring them close. Plant your feet. Exhale as you stand. Pivot with your feet rather than twisting while you hold them. These patterns keep joy and safety together.

Nutrition supports every session. Protein at each meal gives your muscles the building blocks they need to adapt. Calcium rich foods and vitamin D support the mineral side of bone. Magnesium and K2 play their quiet roles. Hydration keeps energy steady. A small snack with protein and carbohydrate before training can help if you feel low on fuel. A meal after training supports recovery. Supplements can fill gaps but they do not replace food.

How will you know your plan is working. You will feel steadier when you walk. You will get up from chairs with less effort. You will carry bags closer to your body without thinking. You will notice fewer near stumbles. These are early signs. Over time your training log will show more repetitions or slightly heavier loads done with the same calm form. When you repeat a DEXA on the same machine after a sensible interval, you may see stability or small gains. Celebrate all of these markers. They mean your bones are hearing the message.

The destination is not a perfect number. It is a body that moves with trust. Training that builds bone is simple, respectful, and steady. Choose patterns that load the hips and spine. Progress in small steps. Keep your spine long. Breathe during effort. Pair your sessions with food that supports change and with home habits that reduce falls. This is a path you can follow at any age. It brings realistic gains and a life that stays open.

Chapter 11

Weights, Bands, and Bodyweight: What Works and How Much Load Is Right

People often ask which tool is best for bones. The honest answer is that all three can help in different ways. Bodyweight teaches positions and builds control. Bands create smooth resistance and are friendly on joints. Weights deliver the strongest signal to the hips and spine when used with good form. The art is to match the tool to your current level and then progress so that your body keeps adapting without fear.

Begin with bodyweight when you are learning patterns or returning after time away. Sit to stands from a safe chair rehearse the squat pattern and load the hips and thighs. A hip hinge to touch a box or the back of a couch teaches you to bend from the hips while keeping a long spine. Wall push ups and gentle rows against a door frame wake up the upper body while you practice steady breathing. Bodyweight work shows you how alignment feels when nothing pulls you off balance. It sets the stage for heavier signals later.

Bands are the next step for many people. A loop around the legs teaches the hips to resist inward collapse during squats and step ups. A long band anchored at chest height allows rows and presses that build the back and shoulders while your trunk stays quiet. Bands are easy to carry on trips, so routines survive travel. They also let you adjust resistance by stepping farther from the anchor or by choosing a thicker band. For bone density, bands are excellent for learning and for maintenance, yet they often fall short as the only tool when the goal is to raise DEXA numbers at the hip and spine. Think of them as partners to weights rather than replacements.

Weights include dumbbells, kettlebells, barbells, and machines. They allow you to place clear load through the skeleton. A goblet squat with a kettlebell held close teaches you to stay tall and to use your legs. A deadlift pattern with a weight near your shins teaches the hinge and strengthens the back of the body. A leg press or a chest press on a machine guides the path so you can focus on effort and breath. Machines can feel reassuring in the beginning because they stabilize you while you learn to produce force. Free weights add a balance challenge and transfer well to daily tasks. Both have a role. Choose the version that helps you move well today and build confidence.

How much load is right depends on control, breath, and the feeling of effort at the end of a set. A simple way to judge is to ask yourself how many more smooth repetitions you could do when the set ends. If the answer is two or three, the load is probably in a productive range. If you could do ten more, the signal is too small for bone. If you could not complete the set with steady posture, the load is too high. You can also notice your breath. During a good set you can exhale on the effort and inhale on the return without holding your breath or straining your neck. If your breath becomes choppy, pause and reset. This kind of self check keeps training safe and effective without complicated math.

The spine cares about how you shape forces as much as how heavy the weight is. Keep your head tall and your ribs gently stacked over your pelvis. Hinge from the hips rather than rounding from the waist. Bring loads close to your body so the lever is short. Move with control rather than speed. Exhale as you stand or press. Avoid twisting while you hold weight. These rules sound simple because they are. They are also powerful protectors of the tiny beams inside the vertebrae.

Progression can be small and steady. When a weight feels easy for your planned sets on two sessions in a row, choose the next heavier option. If weights increase in big jumps, you can add repetitions first, then move up a size later. You can also slow the lowering phase slightly to increase challenge without adding load. Rotate movements across the week so that hips, thighs, back, and upper body all receive attention. Two or three focused sessions each week give your bones a regular message. Between sessions, walk and practice balance so that your fall risk drops as your strength rises.

Soreness can be a normal sign that tissues are adapting, especially when you start. It should feel like stiffness or a mild ache in the muscles and it should fade over a day or two. Sharp pain, joint catching, sudden pulling, or pain that makes you change how you move is a reason to stop and reassess. If you are unsure, reduce the weight, improve alignment, and try again on another day. Recovery habits such as protein at each meal, enough fluid, and calm sleep help your body respond to training.

If you have a history of vertebral fracture, the same tools still apply with careful timing. Early on, bodyweight patterns and bands are your friends.

Practice hip hinges to a safe target, sit to stands from a higher chair, gentle rows, and supported step ups. As symptoms settle and you receive clearance, add modest weights. Keep the load close, the spine long, and the breath smooth. Introduce heavier work later when your posture stays tall across every repetition and the day after training feels normal. Your progress is not a race. It is a series of steady steps back to full living.

Walking has a place in the plan but cannot carry it alone. It is excellent for heart health, mood, and general energy. It maintains bone more than it builds it, mainly at the lower leg rather than the hip and spine. Pair your walks with strength work so that bones see both impact and loading. Short brisk segments on level ground can add a power element if your joints are comfortable, yet they do not replace the need to lift.

People often worry that weights are dangerous. The truth is that poor technique under any load is risky, and good technique under a right sized load is safe. Start where you are. Learn shapes with bodyweight. Use bands to build control. Add weights when positions feel natural. Ask for a session with a coach or therapist who understands osteoporosis if that is available. If you train at home, choose simple movements and keep the area clear so you can set weights down safely. Place lighter dumbbells on a table rather than the floor to reduce bending. Use a stable chair or countertop for balance when needed.

Travel and busy schedules do not have to break your plan. On the road, keep bands in your bag and find a chair for sit to stands and hinges. In hotel gyms, choose machines that match your home patterns. If you miss a few days, start again with one lighter session and then return to your normal loads. Consistency over time beats perfection in any single week.

Nutrition makes every tool work better. A serving of protein at breakfast, lunch, and dinner gives your muscles what they need to adapt. Calcium rich foods and vitamin D support the mineral side of bone. Magnesium and K2 play supportive roles. If appetite is lower after training, a simple yogurt, a glass of fortified soy milk, or a small sandwich can start recovery before a larger meal.

You will know you have chosen the right tool and load when daily tasks feel easier and your confidence returns. Standing from a chair becomes smooth. Carrying groceries feels organized. Lifting a suitcase into a trunk happens without a second thought because you bring it close, plant your feet, and exhale as you move. These are the wins that matter. Over months your log will show steady increases. At your next scan, numbers may hold steady or rise modestly. That stability is often the result of many small choices done well.

In the end, the best tool is the one you will use with care. Bodyweight teaches your body the map. Bands keep the map active and travel well. Weights draw bolder lines that bones can read. Choose a simple path, move in small steps, and let your bones hear a clear message week after week. This is how you build strength you can trust.

Chapter 12

Walking, Yoga, and Pilates: What Helps, What to Modify, What to Avoid

Walking, yoga, and Pilates are three popular ways to move. Many people enjoy them because they fit easily into life and do not require much equipment. After an osteoporosis diagnosis you may wonder whether they are still safe. The good news is that all three can support strong bones and better balance when you use them with care. This chapter explains what each practice offers, what to change, and which shapes to skip so that your spine and hips stay protected.

Start with walking because it is the most common habit. Walking supports heart health, mood, and energy. It keeps joints moving and helps you maintain a healthy weight. For bone density walking maintains more than it builds, especially at the spine. That does not mean walking loses its place. It means you pair it with strength training so that your bones receive a clearer signal. Think of walking as the base of your movement week. Choose routes that are even and well lit when you want to walk briskly. If your joints are comfortable, add short segments where you pick up the pace on level ground. These bursts wake up the muscles that steady your hips and pelvis. They also train your reaction time, which reduces falls. If your neighborhood has uneven sidewalks, ease into speed only after the first minutes when your body has read the surface. Shoes with good grip and a secure heel make a real difference. If vision changes make curbs hard to read, slow down near changes in height and keep your eyes level so you can see the edge early.

Some people ask whether walking with poles is helpful. Light poles or a well fitted cane can add stability on uneven ground. They allow you to keep a long spine while you step over cracks or roots. The tool does not mean you are weak. It means you have chosen stability so that you can stay active outdoors. If you live where winter is icy, simple traction cleats that slip over shoes can turn slippery days into safe days.

Yoga is a broad world that ranges from very gentle to very intense. The benefits include flexibility, breath control, body awareness, and calm focus. These help posture and balance, which lower fall risk. The key is to choose shapes that respect the spine. Deep forward bends that round the back under load can stress the tiny beams inside the vertebrae. Quick roll downs and sit ups that curl the spine with force are also risky for many people with low bone density. Fast twists with load are not friendly either. What works better is a neutral spine with length from head to tail. You can fold at the hips while keeping your back long. You can twist gently while you stand tall and breathe. You can build flexibility in the hips, shoulders, and ankles while the back stays quiet. A teacher who understands osteoporosis can help you adapt any class. Let them know you prefer long lines, slow entries and exits, and no deep rounding of the spine.

If you enjoy sun salutations, you can modify them to keep the long back you want. Step back to a plank rather than jumping. Lower your knees for support when you move toward the floor. Rise with a long spine rather than a quick roll up. When you reach toward your toes, place your hands on blocks or a chair so that your spine stays long and your hips do the bending. When you twist, imagine length before rotation and move within a small comfortable range. These changes keep the benefits while reducing the risk to the vertebrae.

Pilates focuses on control of the center of the body. It teaches how to align the ribs over the pelvis and how to move arms and legs while the trunk stays steady. This is valuable for spine protection in daily life. Classical Pilates includes many exercises that roll the spine segment by segment. People with low bone density should avoid those shapes. You do not need them to gain strength and control. Choose versions that keep a neutral spine on the mat or equipment. Think about a long back with the rib cage heavy and the pelvis quiet. Movements like a supported bridge where you lift your hips while keeping the spine long teach your hips and back to share load. Leg slides and heel taps train the lower abdominals without curling the spine. Rows and presses with small weights or springs build the upper back while posture stays tall.

Breathing patterns support both yoga and Pilates. Many people lift the chest and arch the back when they inhale. This can push the ribs forward and strain the spine. Practice breathing that expands into the sides and back of the rib cage. Place your hands on the lower ribs and feel them widen on the inhale and return on the exhale. Use this breath during transitions. Exhale as you stand from the floor. Exhale as you press a weight away. Calm breath keeps your trunk engaged and your neck relaxed.

People often ask what to avoid in simple terms. Avoid deep forward bends that round the upper or lower back, especially when you are lifting or holding a load. Avoid quick roll downs that move one vertebra at a time under force. Avoid rapid twisting while bent forward or while holding weight. Avoid extreme end range positions that you cannot control. Replace these with hip hinges where your back stays long, gentle twists done while tall, and slow transitions with steady breath. These changes are not about fear. They are about shaping forces so that your bones receive friendly signals.

How do these practices fit with weights and bands. They fit well when you see them as partners. A week that includes two short strength sessions and several walks builds bone and heart health together. One or two yoga or Pilates sessions teach alignment and control that you can use during lifts and during daily tasks. If you have time for only one, choose the practice that feels most calming and useful in your life right now. Consistency beats complexity.

If you have had a vertebral fracture, you can still enjoy walking, yoga, and Pilates with timing and guidance. Early on, keep walks short and gentle. Let pain guide your distance. Choose yoga shapes that keep a long spine and skip forward folds for now. In Pilates stay with neutral spine work. As healing progresses and your clinician clears you, add a little more range. The moment to progress is when your posture stays tall during the whole session and the next day feels normal. If a movement creates sharp pain or a sense of instability, stop and choose a simpler shape. Recovery is not a straight line. It is a path with many steady steps.

Travel can support all three practices. Walking is built in at airports and city visits. Stretching at a hotel with a towel as a strap can replace floor forward bends. Short Pilates style sessions in a room can keep your spine aware of alignment. If your schedule is full, choose five minutes of breath and posture work before bed. Consistency over the week is more important than the length of any single session.

Nutrition helps these activities feel good and work better. Protein at each meal supports muscle repair. Calcium rich foods and vitamin D support bone. Hydration keeps energy steady and helps with balance, especially when you stand up after sitting. If you train with weights on some days and do yoga or Pilates on others, keep meals steady so your tissues have the building blocks they need.

You will know you are on the right track when walking feels smoother, when you stand taller without effort, and when you no longer think about how to pick up a bag because your hips hinge and your breath guides you. You may still choose to avoid certain shapes in yoga or Pilates because you prefer safety. That is a wise and confident choice. The goal is not to perform a specific pose. The goal is a body that moves through daily life with control.

To sum up in plain words, walking is healthy and keeps you moving, yet it needs the support of strength work if you want to change bone density. Yoga and Pilates help posture, balance, and breath when you keep your back long and avoid deep rounding and fast twisting. Modify shapes, slow transitions, and choose teachers who welcome questions. With these choices you can keep the practices you love and protect your bones at the same time.

Chapter 13

Sports and Hobbies: How to Play Safely and Confidently

Life after an osteoporosis diagnosis should include the activities you love. Sports and hobbies bring joy, friendship, and a sense of identity. You do not have to give them up. You may need to adjust how you play so that forces on your spine and hips stay friendly. This chapter shows you how to think about risk, how to warm up, how to shape techniques, and how to return to favorite activities with confidence.

Begin with a simple idea. Risk is not the same for everyone and it is not the same for every sport. Your personal risk depends on your bone density and quality, your history of fractures, your balance, your strength, your vision, your medications, and your environment. The sport's risk depends on speed, impact, twisting, and the chance of falls or collisions. When you match your personal risk to the sport's profile, you can make smart adjustments rather than broad bans. This is empowering because it keeps you in the game with a plan.

Warm up matters even more now. Before any session spend a few minutes waking up your hips, shoulders, and breath. Stand tall and take slow inhales that expand your sides and back. Hinge at the hips with a long spine as if closing a drawer. Practice a few sit to stands from a safe height. Take short steps and feel your feet press the ground under the heel, arch, and big toe. Add gentle rows with a light band to wake the upper back. These simple moves set your alignment before play begins.

If you enjoy tennis or pickleball, you can keep playing with smart spacing and posture. The main risks come from sudden forward bends to reach low balls and from twisting while rounded. Stay a little farther back so the ball rises to a height where you can reach with your legs and a tall spine. Bend your knees and hinge from your hips rather than rounding your back. Rotate your whole body with the shot rather than twisting through a flexed spine. Split step softly so your feet are ready, and choose shoes with a grippy sole. Practice footwork drills that move you with small steps rather than lunges from a rounded back. During serves and overheads, keep your ribs stacked over your pelvis and let your legs drive the motion.

If you love golf, spine friendly technique is possible. Many players round at address and then swing from a flexed, rotated position. Choose a neutral posture with a long back and a small hip hinge. Let your ribs settle so your chest does not flare. Turn around your hips and mid back rather than cranking from the low back. Shorten your backswing a little if needed to keep control. Use longer clubs or adjust grip if you tend to reach and round. Warm up with gentle hip hinges and slow practice swings that keep your head tall. Walk the course if balance and endurance allow, or use a push cart rather than carrying a heavy bag. When lifting the bag into a car, bring it close and exhale as you move.

Cycling protects joints and builds stamina. On a road bike or spin bike, set the handlebar height so that your back stays long and your hips hinge rather than rounding. Keep your elbows slightly bent and your shoulders relaxed. If the saddle is too high, your hips rock and your low back strains. If it is too low, your knees and hips feel compressed and your power drops. Ask a professional for a basic fit or use simple guides to adjust seat height to a position where your knee has a small bend at the bottom of the pedal stroke. On outdoor rides be cautious with gravel, wet leaves, and traffic. A stable hybrid or upright bike can feel safer than an aggressive racing position. Helmets are non negotiable.

Swimming is friendly to the spine when you keep length and avoid rapid twisting. Freestyle can work well if you rotate the whole body as a unit and keep the neck long. Breaststroke can stress the low back if the kick is too wide or the head lifts too high. Keep the kick narrow and let your chest rise with your head so the neck does not jam. Backstroke supports posture and may feel especially good. Water walking and gentle water aerobics add resistance with low impact and are helpful when land based training feels sore.

Dancing brings joy and balance training in one. Choose styles and tempos that let you keep a tall posture and controlled steps. Quick deep dips or dramatic back bends may not be friendly to vertebrae. Partner dances can be safe when communication is clear and steps are predictable. Solo classes with mirrored walls help you monitor posture. Flexible shoes and smooth floors reduce stumbles.

Hiking offers fresh air and varied movement. Start with even trails and build your tolerance before tackling roots and rocks. Poles add stability and let your arms share the work on hills. Keep your backpack light and close to your body. When you step down from a rock or a ledge, keep your spine long and bend at the hips and knees. If you need to cross streams or uneven logs, slow down and place your feet carefully rather than reaching from a rounded back.

Gardening is a favorite hobby that can be adapted. The common risks are long periods of bending and twisting while lifting bags or soil. Use a small bench or pad so you can work closer to the ground without rounding. Bring pots up to a table to avoid lifting from the floor. Break heavy bags into smaller containers that you can hold close. Hinge from the hips with a long back when you reach into raised beds. Take breaks to stand tall, breathe, and walk a few steps to reset your posture.

Strength sports can fit too with the right approach. If you enjoy the gym, machines provide a guided path for presses, rows, and leg work that loads bone with control. Free weights add a balance challenge and transfer well to daily tasks when you master form. You can learn a kettlebell deadlift with a long spine and the bell close to your body. You can squat to a target that lets you keep control. You can press weights while keeping your ribs quiet and your breath smooth. If you compete or enjoy heavier lifts, work with a coach who understands osteoporosis so that progression remains safe.

Many people ask how to judge whether a sport is worth the risk. A good test is to notice how your spine feels during and after the activity and to watch your movement patterns. If the sport encourages you to move with a long back, to use your legs, and to rotate your whole body rather than twisting through a rounded spine, it is likely friendly. If the sport rewards quick forward bends, fast twisting under load, or frequent falls, adjust the way you play or consider a different version. For example, choose doubles rather than singles in racket sports to reduce court coverage speed. Choose groomed slopes and slower turns if you ski and avoid icy days. Choose a kayak with a supportive seat back if you paddle.

If you have had a vertebral fracture, your return to sports is stepwise. Early on focus on posture, walking, and gentle strength. As pain settles and your clinician clears you, add controlled drills that mirror your sport. Tennis players practice footwork and short strokes with a tall spine. Golfers practice address and half swings. Hikers build tolerance on smooth trails before uneven ones. Cyclists ride indoors on a stable bike before outdoor routes. Confidence returns when your body experiences success in small doses.

Travel and busy schedules can support your hobbies when you plan. Pack a light band for warm ups and a small ball for gentle soft tissue work. Choose accommodations near parks or paths. If you will be lifting suitcases, treat those lifts with the same care you use in the gym. Bring loads close. Plant your feet. Exhale as you move. Pivot rather than twist. These patterns keep your back safe so you can enjoy the main event.

Nutrition, hydration, and sleep complete the picture. A serving of protein at each meal supports muscle repair after active days. Calcium rich foods and vitamin D support bone. Water helps attention and balance during play. Sleep restores reaction time and mood. If supplements are part of your plan, keep them consistent while traveling so that energy and recovery stay steady.

The goal is not to remove all risk. The goal is to live fully with eyes open. Sports and hobbies shape your identity and give meaning to your week. Keep them by adjusting technique, improving posture and balance, and building strength. Ask for coaching when needed. Start small, celebrate wins, and progress at a pace that respects your body. With these steps you can play safely and confidently for many years.

Chapter 14

Lifting Loved Ones: Holding and Carrying Grandchildren Safely

Few joys match the feeling of a child running into your arms. After an osteoporosis diagnosis many people worry that this moment is over. It is not. You can hold and carry grandchildren safely when you shape how you lift, how you stand, and how you breathe. This chapter gives you clear steps to protect your spine and hips while keeping family life warm and active.

Start with a simple picture of a safe lift. Keep your spine long, bring the child close to your body, plant your feet, and use your legs. Distance is the enemy because it makes the load feel heavier to your back. Closeness is your friend because it shortens the lever and lets your hips and thighs do the work. Before you lift, take a calm breath out to set gentle support around your middle. Then move with smooth control rather than speed.

Approach the lift like a small dance. Stand with your feet about hip width and feel the floor under your heels, arches, and big toes. Hinge from your hips and bend your knees enough to reach the child without rounding your back. Slide your arms around the child and pull them close to your chest or shoulder before you rise. Keep your chin slightly tucked so your neck stays long. Exhale as you stand and imagine pushing the floor away with your feet. If you need to turn, take small steps to face the new direction rather than twisting while you hold the child. These actions protect the tiny beams inside your vertebrae.

Set up the environment so that safe choices are the easy ones. When possible, meet the child at a higher surface like a couch edge or a bench so you lift over a shorter distance. Ask older toddlers to climb onto your lap or onto a low step and then guide them up with your hands so you are not reaching from the floor. If you use a stroller or car seat, bring it up onto a stable surface before you secure straps or lift it to the car. Avoid leaning into the back seat with a rounded spine while holding the seat at arm's length. Slide the seat close, plant your feet, and pivot your whole body as you place it.

How long can you carry a child and how heavy is safe. The answer depends on your strength, your posture control, and whether you have pain. A practical rule is to carry for shorter distances and set the child down often rather than holding for long periods. Change sides regularly to share the work between both arms and to keep your posture from drifting. If you notice your ribs flaring, your low back arching, or your head sliding forward, it is time to rest. You can sit with the child on your lap and keep the connection without the load.

Lifting is easier when your legs, hips, and back are trained for it. Strength training gives you the reserve to handle family moments without strain. Practice sit to stands from a chair while keeping a long spine and exhaling as you stand. Practice hip hinges with a weight held close to your body so the pattern becomes automatic. Practice carries with a grocery bag or a light kettlebell held in front of your chest. These drills mirror real life and teach your body to organize under load. Over time the reserve you build shows up as calm confidence when a child jumps into your arms.

What if you have had a vertebral fracture. You can still return to lifting, but the path is gradual. During the early healing phase focus on posture, breathing, short walks, and gentle leg strength. Ask for help with lifting and carrying. As pain settles and your clinician clears you, begin with supported holds where a child sits on your lap while you keep a long spine. Then practice rising from a chair while holding a small pillow to your chest to simulate a close load. Later add light carries with an object before you lift a child again. The signal that you are ready is a combination of steady posture, no sharp pain during or after practice, and a normal feeling the next day. The timeline is personal and there is no rush.

What about newborns and car seats. New babies are light but the positions around them can be tricky. When you lift a car seat from the ground, squat close, slide your hand under the handle near the child's head rather than reaching far away, and keep the seat close to your body as you rise. If the seat feels awkward, ask another adult to hold the base steady while you guide the seat into place. When you lean over a crib, step close and keep your spine long. Lower from your hips and knees. If the crib rail is high, place a small step for your feet so you do not reach with straight legs and a rounded back.

Playtime can be active without risky shapes. Choose games that keep the child close to your center. March in place together. Sit on the floor with your back against a couch and roll a ball back and forth. Kneel on one knee to be at eye level rather than bending from the waist. If you like to lift a toddler into the air, do it while seated with the child facing you and move through small ranges. Keep your ribs stacked over your pelvis so your low back does not arch. If you feel uncertain, switch to games where your legs do the work and your spine stays quiet.

Getting a child in and out of a car is a common challenge. Stand close to the seat, place one foot in the car to bring your hips nearer, and keep the child close to your chest as you pivot both feet to face the seat. Lower by bending your hips and knees instead of twisting. To lift out, reverse the move. Bring the child to your chest, plant both feet facing the door, and rise with an exhale. If your car is low, consider a small cushion to raise your seat or park where you can open doors fully to reduce awkward angles.

Travel adds moving parts, but the same principles apply. Use wheeled bags so that your hands are free for railings and for the child's hand. Ask for aisle seats on planes and trains so you can stand easily. In airports, use elevators rather than escalators when you carry a child or a stroller. If you need to place a bag in an overhead bin, rest it first on the seat back to shorten the lift and use both hands with a long spine. Plan breaks for walking and stretching so that fatigue does not push you into rushed movements.

Nutrition and energy change how lifting feels. A body that is well fed handles load more calmly. Protein at each meal helps your muscles adapt to training and recover after active days with the family. Calcium rich foods and vitamin D support bone. Hydration keeps attention and balance sharp when you move with a child in your arms. These quiet supports show up when you reach, stand, and pivot under load.

Pain and warning signs deserve attention. Normal muscle effort feels like work during a lift and mild stiffness the day after. Sharp pain in the spine, a sudden catching feeling, or pain that changes how you move is a reason to stop and reset. If symptoms persist, speak with your clinician. Adjust the size of the child you lift, the distance you carry, and the surfaces you choose. Meet at couches rather than the floor. Ask children to climb to your lap when they can. Use a stroller for longer walks.

Grandparents often ask whether lifting loved ones could undo the gains from medication or training. The answer is reassuring. When done with good form and reasonable loads, family lifting sits well inside a safe envelope and does not cancel progress. In fact, the same patterns you practice in the gym protect you at home. Long spine. Load close. Hips and legs doing the work. Calm breathing during effort. These habits turn a moment of joy into a movement that builds trust in your body.

If you prefer not to lift at all, connection does not disappear. Sitting on a couch and reading together, walking hand in hand, building blocks at a table, and gentle dancing with the child standing on your feet all create closeness without heavy loads. You can still be the lap, the safe arms, and the steady presence in the room.

Holding and carrying grandchildren safely is not about strength alone. It is about alignment, breath, environment, and patience. Practice the small dance of a safe lift when life is quiet so it is ready when a child runs to you. Ask for help on hard days. Choose positions that bring the child close and keep your spine long. With these choices you protect your bones and keep family moments open and joyful.

Chapter 15

Travel with Ease: Planning, Packing, Moving Without Risk

You do not have to stop traveling after an osteoporosis diagnosis. You can still visit family, explore new places, and enjoy weekends away. Safe travel is about shaping small choices before and during the trip so that your spine and hips see friendly forces. With a bit of planning, packing, and mindful movement, the journey becomes part of the joy rather than a source of worry.

Begin with planning because it sets the tone. Choose routes and schedules that reduce rushing. If possible, allow extra time for transfers so you can walk without hurrying. Request aisle seats so standing and walking breaks are easy. If stairs are common in your destination, look for lodging with elevators or ground floor rooms. Read hotel or rental descriptions with your spine in mind. Showers with a ledge for balance, beds at a comfortable height, and good lighting make a difference after a long day. Think about the kind of walking surface you will meet. Old towns with cobblestones or trails with roots are beautiful, but they change how you move. Knowing this in advance helps you pack shoes with grip and plan your pace.

Packing shapes the loads you carry. Light bags are safer bags. Choose a suitcase with four wheels that rolls beside you so your arm stays close to your body and your spine stays long. Pack a small day bag that fits on your back rather than one shoulder so your hands remain free for rails and doors. Spread weight across two smaller bags instead of one heavy case if that keeps each lift friendly. Place heavy items near the wheels and close to the handle so lifts are shorter. Keep medications, snacks, water, and any supplement you use in a small pouch you can reach without digging. The goal is calm movement, not perfect organization.

Lifting luggage is a common worry and a real place to practice safe patterns. When you lift a bag from the floor, stand close and plant your feet. Hinge from your hips and bend your knees to reach the handle while keeping your back long. Exhale as you stand and keep the bag near your body. To place a bag in a car trunk, rest it on the edge first to shorten the lever, then slide it in rather than swinging it from a distance. To pull a suitcase off a carousel, step close, bring the handle to your chest, and pivot your feet to face the direction you want to go. Overhead bins on planes deserve special care. If a bag is heavy, ask for help. If you place it yourself, put it first on the seat back to reduce the lift, then use both hands to guide it up while your spine stays long. There is no prize for lifting alone. There is a win in arriving with a happy back.

Airports and stations add many transitions. Move as if you were training. Keep a tall posture, let your arms swing freely, and look a few steps ahead to read the floor. Use elevators when you carry bags or when escalators feel crowded. On escalators, hold the rail and keep your bag in front rather than behind so you can see it and keep it close. On moving walkways, step on and off with a calm pace and eyes level. If crowds make you tense, pause at the side for a breath and wait for a clear lane. Attention is a quiet safety tool.

On planes and trains, long sitting can make the back feel stiff. You can help your body with small routines that fit the space. Sit tall with your ribs stacked over your pelvis and your feet grounded. Let your breath expand your sides and back rather than lifting your chest. Every half hour, slide to the edge of the seat, hinge forward with a long spine, and stand if space allows. If you cannot stand, gently press your feet into the floor and imagine lengthening your head away from your seat back for a few breaths. Roll your shoulders slowly and let your neck turn within a small comfortable range. These actions nourish the tissues that hold you tall.

Hotels and rentals vary in height and layout. When you arrive, do a quick safety scan. Notice light switches, bath mats, and the path between bed and bathroom at night. If the bed is very low, use extra pillows to make getting out easier. If the shower floor is slippery, place a towel at the entrance and move slowly. When you reach into low drawers or mini fridges, hinge at the hips and keep items close to your body as you stand. If a safe kettlebell deadlift pattern is part of your training at home, your body will recognize this hinge automatically and protect your back.

Food and hydration support travel just as they support training. A steady supply of protein at meals helps you handle lifting and long walks. Calcium rich choices and vitamin D keep the mineral side of bone covered. Carry water and sip regularly so blood pressure stays steady when you stand. Low fuel and low fluids invite dizziness and rushed movement. A piece of fruit and a yogurt, a small sandwich, or a handful of nuts can steady you during connections.

Walking tours and museum days often mean many hours on your feet. Pace yourself as if you were doing intervals. Build in short seated breaks before you need them and use these pauses to reset your posture. Place both feet on the floor, breathe into your sides and back, and let your shoulders settle. When you stand again, hinge from your hips, push through your feet, and exhale. If the ground is uneven, shorten your stride for the first minutes while your body reads the surface. Poles can help on trails or in hilly towns and are a sign of wisdom, not weakness.

If you are traveling with family, plan roles that match strengths. Someone can handle overhead bins. Someone can guide toddlers by the hand. Someone can read signs and tickets so you can focus on safe steps. If you carry a child, keep them close to your chest, plant your feet before you stand, and pivot rather than twist as you turn toward the seat or stroller. You will recognize these patterns from the chapter on lifting loved ones. The same moves protect you in stations and on platforms.

Mobility aids and services can turn stressful parts of travel into calm ones. Many airports offer assistance from curb to gate. Trains and ferries have staff who can help with steps and bags. Using these options is not giving up. It is choosing a smooth path so you can save energy for the parts of the trip you love. If you prefer to move on your own, pick times of day when stations are less crowded and lines are shorter. Choose routes with fewer transfers even if the total time is a bit longer.

People often ask whether travel interrupts training. It does not have to. Two short sessions in your room each week can maintain your patterns. Sit to stands from a chair, hip hinges with a backpack held close, supported rows with a band anchored in a door, and balance practice near a wall keep your system tuned. Walk on most days and carry groceries or water close to your body. Your bones like regular signals more than perfect equipment.

Pain or warning signs deserve attention on the road. Normal effort feels like a steady work during lifts and a mild stiffness after long walks. Sharp pain, sudden catching, numbness, or weakness that changes how you move is a reason to stop, rest, and consider medical care. If you have a history of vertebral fracture, keep the early healing rules in mind. Avoid deep forward bends with load and fast twists under pressure. Choose seats and surfaces that let you keep a long spine. Ask for help without hesitation.

The picture that emerges is encouraging. Travel asks for the same friendly patterns you use at home. Long spine. Load close. Calm breath on effort. Eyes level to read the floor. Hands free when possible. Light bags and wheels. Breaks that reset your posture. Protein, calcium rich foods, and water to support energy and balance. With these choices your trips become smoother. Airports become practice grounds rather than obstacles. Stations become familiar. Your bones and muscles adapt to the rhythms of movement instead of feeling threatened by them.

A diagnosis does not shrink your map. It gives you a reason to plan with care so that you can keep exploring. When you travel with intention, you collect experiences rather than injuries. You return home tired in the best way, with stories to tell and a body that feels trusted. That is the marker of a successful trip

Chapter 16

Training After a Vertebral Fracture: When You Can Lift Again

A vertebral fracture can shake your confidence. Many people fear that movement will make things worse. The truth is kinder. Healing needs calm time at first, then gentle motion, then measured strength. Training is part of recovery. It helps pain settle, posture return, and daily life feel normal again. This chapter explains what to expect week by week, how to move safely, when load can return, and how to read your own green lights and red flags.

First, a simple picture of healing. A fresh vertebral fracture is like a bruise inside the bone. In the early phase the goal is comfort and protection while the body lays down new tissue. Pain is a guide. Sharp spikes of pain mean you have asked for too much. Dull stiffness that eases with small movements is common and often a sign that gentle activity is helping. Your clinician will confirm the diagnosis, check for other causes of pain, and advise on bracing if needed. Some people wear a soft or rigid brace for a short time. Others do not. Follow the plan you are given. Braces can reduce pain while you learn safer patterns, but they are not a long term solution. Muscles must return to work.

During the early weeks focus on positions that feel supported. Lying on your side with a pillow between your knees often calms symptoms. Lying on your back with a small pillow under your knees can help some people. Roll in and out of bed like a log so your spine stays long. Sit on a chair with your hips slightly higher than your knees and place both feet on the floor. Let your ribs soften so your chest does not flare forward. Breathe into your sides and back. This style of breath spreads pressure and helps you relax. Short walks around the home keep circulation moving. Keep steps slow and smooth. Pain that fades after these walks is a good sign.

Posture practice begins almost at once. Think tall and relaxed rather than stiff. Imagine a line from the crown of your head to your tailbone. Let your shoulders rest wide and your ribs settle over your pelvis. When you stand from a chair, bring your feet under you, lean forward with a long back, and exhale as you rise. These small details protect the tiny beams inside the vertebrae and become automatic with practice.

As pain settles, usually over several weeks, gentle strength can begin. The goal is to wake up hips, legs, and the mid back while keeping the injured area quiet. Start with isometric holds where muscles work without motion. Press your feet into the floor as if to grow taller. Hold for a few breaths and relax. Place your hands against a wall and press lightly as if to start a push up while your spine stays long. Do supported standing rows with a light band anchored at chest height. Think of your shoulder blades gliding toward your spine as you pull. Stop if you feel sharp pain or if your breath becomes choppy. Smooth breaths mean the load is friendly.

The next step is controlled movement with light resistance. Practice sit to stands from a higher chair. Touch down and stand up with calm breath. Practice hip hinges where you reach your hips back toward a wall while your back stays long. Touch a box or the back of a couch, then return to standing. Add supported step ups on a low platform and hold a railing or counter for balance. These drills teach your body to share load across hips and legs instead of asking the spine to bend and twist.

When can you lift again. The first answer is when pain at rest is calm, when daily tasks feel steady, and when your clinician clears you. The second answer is when your posture remains long during practice and the day after training feels normal. Many people can begin lifting light external loads within several weeks. Some need longer. The timeline is individual, and that is normal. The plan is to add load in small steps and to keep the weight close to your body. A light kettlebell or dumbbells held at your chest are often friendlier than a long bar that sits far from your center.

Start with a load that feels almost easy. Hold a kettlebell or a bag of books close to your chest and practice a few hip hinges to a target, then a few short carries while you walk tall. Exhale as you stand or step. If the session feels steady and you feel normal the next day, repeat it. When two sessions in a row feel easy, add a little more weight or a few more repetitions. This slow progression is how bones and tissues adapt. There is no need to chase numbers. The marker of success is control.

Which movements belong in your program. Hinge based patterns load the hips while protecting the spine. A squat to a box set at a safe height teaches you to share work across both legs. A supported deadlift pattern with a kettlebell held close teaches a long back and strong hips. A step up to a stable platform trains balance and leg strength. Rows and presses for the upper body build the back and shoulders that help posture. Avoid deep forward bends with load and fast twisting under pressure. Replace them with tall positions and slow transitions.

What if you feel nervous. Confidence returns through repetition in safe shapes. Practice in a quiet space with a stable chair or countertop nearby. Set up your environment so that you do not have to rush. Put the phone away. Place the weight on a table rather than the floor so you do not need to bend far to pick it up. Wear shoes that grip and clothing that lets you move. Invite a family member to be present for the first sessions if that calms you. Many people find that the first minutes feel tense and then the body remembers how to move.

People often ask whether walking, yoga, and Pilates help during recovery. Walking is useful from early on because it brings circulation and resets posture. Keep distances short at first and build slowly. Yoga can help when you choose shapes that keep a neutral spine. Skip deep forward folds and quick roll downs. Focus on long lines and gentle twists done while tall. Pilates can teach rib and pelvis control without curling the spine. These practices support your return to lifting but do not replace it.

What about medications and nutrition. If you and your clinician choose a medicine that stabilizes bone biology, that can pair well with training to lower risk. Food supports healing. Protein at each meal provides the building blocks for muscle and the collagen framework in bone. Calcium rich foods and vitamin D support mineralization. Magnesium and K2 play quiet roles in this process. Hydration keeps energy and attention steady so you move with care.

How do you judge progress without waiting for the next scan. Use daily markers. Can you stand from a chair without using your hands. Can you carry a small bag close to your body for the distance you want. Do you feel steadier on uneven ground. Do you have fewer near stumbles. Does your back feel calm the day after training. These answers tell you that your body is adapting. When the time comes to repeat a DEXA or to look at TBS, try to use the same center and positioning so the trend is clear. Numbers will follow function over time.

Return to life tasks in a planned order. First come light household actions with a long spine. Next come short carries with the load close. Then come suitcase lifts and car seat moves done with the patterns you have practiced. Lifting grandchildren returns after these steps feel smooth and after your clinician agrees. Bring the child close. Plant your feet. Exhale as you stand. Pivot rather than twist. Celebrate small wins. They add up.

There will be days when fatigue or stress make form slip. Notice this early and choose simpler shapes. Training while tired is part of life, but the loads on those days should be lower. If you feel sharp pain, sudden catching, new numbness, or weakness, stop and seek advice. These are red flags. Most aches are normal and fade. Respect the ones that do not.

A vertebral fracture is a chapter, not the whole book. Training gives you a way to turn the page. You begin with calm positions and short walks. You add posture practice and breath. You teach your hips and legs to take the strain. You lift light loads close to your body and progress in small steps. You eat to support healing. You rest enough to adapt. The result is a body that trusts movement again. With patience and steady practice, you can lift again and live fully.

Chapter 17

Decade by Decade: Personalized Bone Care and Weekly Plans

Your bones change across a lifetime, but the message they like stays the same. Move often, load wisely, eat to support rebuilding, and organize your days so that falls are less likely. What changes is how you set the dial for each decade. In this chapter you will see how to shape training, nutrition, testing, and daily habits from your thirties through your eighties and beyond. You will also see simple weekly plans that fit real life without turning it upside down.

In your thirties the goal is to protect the peak you have built. Many people live busy years with work and family. Short focused sessions work well. Choose two strength days that load the hips and spine with a long back. Sit to stands, hip hinges, step ups, rows, and presses cover a lot of ground. Add brisk walks on the other days. If you enjoy sports, warm up your hips and shoulders before play. Food should include protein at each meal and calcium rich choices. If you avoid dairy, use fortified plant milks, tofu set with calcium, and small fish with bones. Ask your clinician when a baseline DEXA makes sense if you have risk factors like family history or long term steroid use. If risk is low, you may not need a scan yet. Build habits now so they feel normal later.

In your forties metabolism and recovery can shift. Hormones begin to change for some people. Keep two to three strength sessions each week and add short balance practice at the end of workouts. Stand on one foot near a counter and turn your head gently. Keep your eyes level. Walking remains the foundation. If joints allow, place a few faster minutes into a walk so your muscles learn to respond. Nutrition should include steady protein and calcium. Vitamin D may need attention, especially in winter. If you notice more stiffness, respect warm ups and keep your spine long during all bends and lifts. Travel for work or family can be frequent in this decade. Wheels on bags, loads close to the body, and aisle seats reduce risk and fatigue.

In your fifties many women enter menopause and see a quicker drop in bone density when estrogen falls. Men may also feel slower recovery. This is the decade to take structure seriously. Strength training becomes a non negotiable. Two or three short sessions each week with simple movements done well send a clear signal to bone. Add daily posture moments and short balance drills. Yoga or Pilates can support alignment when you avoid deep forward bends and fast roll downs. Talk with your clinician about a first DEXA if you have not had one, especially if family history or past fractures are part of your story. Review vitamin D and consider K2 and magnesium if your diet is light in those nutrients. Walking stays in the week but does not replace loading for hips and spine. If a sport you love includes quick twists or frequent falls, adjust technique and pace rather than quitting. Confidence comes from skills and planning, not from luck.

In your sixties the plan focuses on steadiness. Keep strength sessions simple and repeatable. Use machines if they help you feel secure. Use free weights if you enjoy them and your form is clear. Choose weights that feel challenging near the end of a set while your breath stays smooth. Keep the load close and your spine long. Add balance practice most days. A minute at the counter while the kettle boils can change how safe you feel on stairs. If you have started a medication for bone, pair it with training and food so outcomes are stronger. If you prefer a non drug path, agree with your clinician on a time frame for training and nutrition, then repeat scans to see trends. Home safety matters more now. Improve light, clear floors, secure rugs, and use grab bars where helpful. These changes prevent everyday fractures as effectively as many pills.

In your seventies strength and balance remain very trainable. People gain muscle at seventy and eighty when they train with care. Sessions can be shorter and still effective. Choose movements that let you keep control. Sit to stands to a higher target, hip hinges with a weight held close, step ups with a support, rows and presses with light dumbbells or bands. Bands travel well and keep patterns alive between weight sessions. Walking stays in the week with routes that are even and well lit. If your vision prescription is old, update it so edges and steps are clear. If a cane or poles add stability outdoors, use them with pride. They keep you moving. Nutrition should prioritize protein, calcium rich foods, and vitamin D because appetite can be variable. Hydration supports attention and balance when you stand.

In your eighties and beyond the theme is trust and simplicity. Keep loading in a friendly range and repeat patterns often. Practice rising from a chair with a long back, carrying a light object close, and stepping up to a safe platform while holding a rail. A few repetitions done most days keep the system awake. Short walks, posture moments, and gentle breath work support energy and mood. If you travel, plan routes with fewer transfers and choose elevators over escalators when you carry bags. Family lifting can continue with the child brought close, feet planted, and breath steady. Joy and safety can live together.

Here are weekly plans that you can use as starting points and adjust to your taste. In your thirties and forties a week might include two strength days and three walking days. Place strength on Monday and Thursday. On those days train your hips and spine with sit to stands, hinges, step ups, and rows, then finish with short balance practice. Walk briskly on Tuesday, Saturday, and a third day that fits your schedule. On other days weave posture and breath moments into chores. In your fifties and sixties keep the same pattern but add a second short balance session on a day you do not lift. If you enjoy yoga or Pilates, place a gentle session on a day after strength to rehearse long spine and controlled breathing. In your seventies and eighties reduce volume and keep frequency. Two shorter strength sessions, three shorter walks, and daily posture checks keep progress steady without fatigue.

Nutrition threads through every decade. Aim for protein at breakfast, lunch, and dinner so muscles adapt to training. Choose calcium rich foods each day and add a simple supplement only if meals fall short. Keep vitamin D steady with food, sun when safe, or a supplement guided by your clinician. Magnesium and K2 can support the plan when your diet is light in those nutrients. Collagen can be a helpful addition if joints feel stiff or if appetite is low, but it does not replace a full protein source. Water keeps blood pressure steady when you stand and helps balance.

Testing needs a calm schedule. If your first DEXA shows low bone mass or osteoporosis, plan the next scan with your clinician based on your risk and treatment choice. Many people repeat a scan after one to two years to see a trend. TBS can add context about spine quality, especially when degenerative changes make interpretation of spine density difficult. Use the same center and positioning when possible so that changes reflect your biology rather than machine differences. Do not chase small shifts. Watch the trend and pair it with how you feel and function.

Common questions appear in each decade and the answers are steady. Can you live normally with osteoporosis. Yes, when you train, fuel, and shape daily habits. Can you play sports. Yes, with technique that keeps a long spine and with warm ups that wake up your hips and shoulders. Can you travel. Yes, with wheels on bags, hands free for rails, and a calm pace. Can you lift grandchildren. Yes, when the load is close, your feet are planted, and you exhale as you stand. Is walking enough. Walking is healthy but does not raise spine density by itself. Pair it with strength work. Are bands enough. Bands are excellent partners and can maintain strength, yet weights often add the stimulus your hips and spine need. Are weights safe. Weights are safe when technique is clear and progress is patient. Can you improve without medications. Many people can improve function and reduce fracture risk with training, nutrition, and fall prevention. If your risk is high or you have a recent fracture, medications can lower risk faster and can be paired with the same habits. How much can density improve. Expect stability or small gains over months and years and celebrate the faster wins in strength, balance, and confidence.

Build your plan with kindness. Choose the simplest actions that you will repeat. Keep a small log so that you see the pattern grow. When life changes, adjust the dial rather than stopping. During busy seasons shorten sessions. During calmer weeks add a set or a walk. Ask your clinician for help when new symptoms appear or when you consider medications. You are not alone in this work. The combination of training, food, safer movement, and supportive care works at any age. It turns a diagnosis into a guide and lets you keep the life you value.

Chapter 18

Partner with Providers, Debunk Myths, and Live Confidently for Life

The strongest bone plan is a partnership. You bring your goals, your daily habits, and your questions. Your healthcare team brings clinical knowledge, test interpretation, and options. Together you choose steps that match your values. This chapter shows you how to work with providers, how to prepare for appointments, how to read advice with a calm mind, and how to clear away common myths that create fear. The destination is confidence that lasts.

Begin with preparation because it changes the quality of every visit. Keep a simple notebook or a note on your phone. Write your main goals in plain words. Fewer fractures. More strength. Easier travel. Being able to lift a grandchild. Add a short list of questions that matter this season. When should I repeat DEXA and TBS. Which exercises are best for me now. Is my calcium intake enough. Do I need a medication or can we try training and food first. Bring a short summary of your weekly routine so your provider sees the work you are doing at home. Include supplements and medicines with amounts and timing. Bring past scan reports and any relevant X ray or MRI notes so trends are easy to read.

During appointments, ask for plain language. It is your right to understand. If a word feels unclear, pause and ask what it means in simple terms. If a risk or benefit is given as a percentage, ask what that could look like in real life. If there are several options, ask which one matches your situation and why. If you are choosing a medication, ask what outcomes you can expect, what side effects to watch for, and how you will review progress. If you prefer a period of non drug care first, suggest a clear time frame for training, food, and fall prevention, then agree on when to rescan. This keeps the plan active.

Your provider is your ally. Share the details that shape care. Mention past fractures, height loss, family history, early menopause, steroid use, stomach or bowel conditions, thyroid issues, and any history of eating disorders. Share sports you love, travel plans, and family roles. A plan that ignores your life will not last. A plan that fits your life will.

Telehealth can work well for follow ups, especially when you need to review test results or adjust supplements. In person visits are helpful for physical exams and for learning movement patterns. If you need guidance on lifting, rows, hinges, and posture, ask for a referral to a physical therapist who understands osteoporosis. One or two sessions can teach you shapes that protect your spine and hips. Many therapists can also help you choose safe starting loads and can build your confidence.

Now let us clear away myths that cause worry.

Myth one says osteoporosis means you must stop living normally. The truth is that you can live fully with smart adjustments. You can play sports with technique that keeps your spine long. You can travel with wheels on bags and hands free for rails. You can lift grandchildren by bringing them close, planting your feet, and exhaling as you stand. You can train with weights that you control. Safety comes from patterns and planning, not from shrinking your life.

Myth two says walking alone will rebuild bone. Walking is healthy for heart, mood, and stamina. It maintains bone more than it builds it, especially at the spine. Pair walking with strength training that loads the hips and back. Add short brisk segments on level ground if your joints allow. This combination sends the signal your skeleton understands.

Myth three says bands are enough for everyone. Bands are excellent for learning control and for travel. They help maintain strength. For many adults they are not enough to raise hip and spine density by themselves. Add progressive external load when positions feel steady. Machines, dumbbells, and kettlebells can all help when used with a long spine and smooth breath.

Myth four says weights are dangerous. Poor technique under any load is risky. Good technique under a right sized load is safe and effective. Choose weights that feel challenging near the end of a set while your posture remains long. Increase in small steps. Stop if you feel sharp pain or dizziness. Ask for coaching if you are unsure. Strength protects you in daily life.

Myth five says you cannot improve without medications. Many people improve function and reduce fracture risk with training, nutrition, and fall prevention. Some people also need medication because risk is high or because a fresh fracture changes the picture. Medicines and habits are not rivals. They are tools you can combine. If you choose a non drug period, agree on a time frame and rescan to check progress.

Myth six says DEXA and TBS numbers tell the whole story. They are important but they are not the only markers that matter. Balance, muscle strength, reaction time, vision, home safety, and how you move each day also shape your risk. Stable numbers plus better function is a strong win. Small numeric gains plus poor balance is not. Track both.

Myth seven says once you start a path you can never change it. Plans evolve. If oral pills upset your stomach, ask about a different form or an infusion. If a schedule feels hard to follow, ask for a plan that fits your week. If a gym makes you tense, use a home program with simple tools. The right plan is one you can repeat.

How do you keep confidence strong between appointments. Notice small wins and write them down. Fewer near stumbles on stairs. A smoother lift into the car trunk. A walk that feels taller. A day of travel without a sore back. These are the results of your training and your choices. They are as real as any number on a page. Share them at your next visit. They help your provider see what works and encourage you to keep going.

If you have a setback, treat it as information, not failure. A week of poor sleep or a new medicine can make you feel unsteady. Reduce loads for a few sessions. Shorten walks. Return to posture drills and calm breath. When energy returns, build back. Recovery is not a straight line for anyone. Your ability to adjust is a sign of strength.

Bring family into your plan if that helps. Share the lifting patterns you use. Ask for help with heavy bags. Choose trips that offer elevators and smooth routes. Teach grandchildren how to climb to your lap. Let friends know you prefer a table that allows you to sit tall. Community turns safety into a shared habit rather than a private worry.

Use simple systems to sustain habits. Place a short training session on two days that already feel predictable. Keep bands or light weights where you will see them. Prepare calcium rich snacks that travel well. Check vitamin D with your clinician during routine blood work. Schedule scans at the same center when possible. Keep shoes with grip near the door. Small anchors support big outcomes.

The last piece is purpose. Changing habits is easier when you remember why. You are building strength to travel, to play, to lift a child, to explore your city, to tend a garden, to dance. You are shaping a life that feels open. Osteoporosis will be part of your story, yet it will not be the author. You write this chapter by chapter with training, food, safer movement, and wise medical choices.

Partner with your providers. Ask for clarity. Respect your values. Debunk myths that feed fear. Practice the patterns that keep your spine long and your steps steady. Eat to support rebuilding. Sleep to recover. Celebrate the improvements you can feel. Over time your confidence will rest not on perfect numbers but on a body that moves with trust. That is living well for life.

Sardine & Lemon Kale Toast (Calcium and Protein Rich)

This savory toast gives your bones a friendly start to the day. Sardines offer calcium and vitamin D because you eat the tiny, soft bones. Kale adds vitamin K and magnesium. Whole grain bread brings extra minerals and fiber that help steady energy. The flavors are bright and comforting, and the method takes only a few minutes.

Ingredients and prep in plain words

Open one small tin of sardines packed in olive oil. Rinse a large handful of kale leaves and strip them from the stems, then slice them thinly. Cut half a lemon and set it aside for juice and zest. Take two slices of sturdy whole grain bread. Keep a small clove of garlic, a spoon of plain Greek yogurt or lactose free yogurt, and a drizzle of extra virgin olive oil nearby. If you enjoy a little heat, keep a pinch of chili flakes ready. Have sea salt and black pepper at hand.

Method explained step by step in sentences

Warm a small pan over medium heat and add a teaspoon of olive oil. Place the sliced kale in the warm pan and let it wilt while you stir slowly. Squeeze in a little lemon juice and add a small pinch of salt. When the kale turns glossy and soft, turn off the heat and set the pan aside. Toast the bread until it is firm enough to hold a topping. While the toast is hot, rub the surface lightly with the cut side of the garlic clove so a gentle flavor stays on the bread. In a small bowl break the sardines into large flakes with a fork and add a spoon of their oil for richness. Add a spoon of yogurt and a few drops of lemon juice, then stir just enough to combine without turning the fish into a paste. Add a little black pepper and, if you like, a pinch of chili. Place the warm kale on the toast, then spoon the sardine mixture over it. Finish with a light drizzle of olive oil and a few strokes of lemon zest so the aroma is fresh.

Why this helps your bones and daily energy

Sardines provide calcium in a form your body can use because the tiny bones are soft and edible. They also bring vitamin D, which helps you absorb calcium from meals. The protein in fish and yogurt supports muscle repair after training and helps you feel steady between meals. Kale adds vitamin K that helps guide calcium into bone tissue and magnesium that quietly supports the mineral matrix. Whole grain bread gives fiber that slows the meal's release of energy and adds small amounts of minerals that contribute across the week. The olive oil and yogurt make the dish satisfying so you are less likely to reach for sweets soon after.

Safe prep and easy variations

If you need a softer texture, mash the sardines more fully with the yogurt and chop the kale very finely so the topping spreads smoothly. If you avoid dairy, use a spoon of hummus or a soy yogurt instead of Greek yogurt. If you need gluten free bread, choose a slice that toasts firmly so it carries the topping without crumbling. For extra calcium you can add a thin layer of tahini under the kale before you add the sardines. If you prefer a milder flavor, use canned salmon with bones in place of sardines and season with lemon and dill.

How to serve and store

Eat the toast soon after assembling so it stays crisp. If you want to pack it for later, keep the elements separate. Carry the sardine mix in a small container on ice, the kale in another container, and toast the bread when you are ready to eat. The sardine mixture keeps well in the fridge for a day. The kale can be wilted ahead and kept chilled for two days. When you are home late from travel or training, this recipe comes together in minutes and gives your bones a useful deposit.

Gentle coaching note

If the idea of sardines is new, start with half a portion on one slice of toast and pair it with a piece of fruit. Notice how steady your energy feels. Meals like this, repeated across the week, support bone health alongside your strength sessions and posture practice.

Calcium Set Tofu Scramble with Sesame Greens

This warm, savory scramble is gentle on digestion and rich in nutrients that support bones and muscles. Using tofu set with calcium gives a reliable dose of absorbable calcium, while sesame and leafy greens add magnesium and vitamin K. The texture is soft enough for sensitive days yet satisfying after training or travel.

Ingredients and prep in plain words

Choose a block of firm tofu that lists calcium sulfate on the label. Rinse a large handful of chopped leafy greens such as kale, chard, or bok choy. Slice half an onion and a small clove of garlic. Keep a thumb of fresh ginger if you enjoy a brighter flavor. Measure a spoon of sesame seeds, a spoon of soy sauce or tamari, a teaspoon of toasted sesame oil, and a teaspoon of olive oil. Have a pinch of turmeric for color and a grind of black pepper. Keep lemon wedges nearby for a fresh finish.

Method explained step by step in sentences

Warm a nonstick or cast iron pan over medium heat and add the olive oil. Soften the onion with a pinch of salt until it turns translucent. Add the garlic and ginger and stir for a minute so the aroma rises without browning. Crumble the tofu into the pan with your hands or a fork. Sprinkle a small pinch of turmeric and a little black pepper over the surface and stir so the color spreads. Let the tofu sit for a minute, then stir again so it develops small golden edges without drying out. Add the chopped greens and a splash of water if the pan looks dry. Stir until the greens wilt and turn glossy. Pour in the soy sauce or tamari and mix to coat everything evenly. Turn off the heat and finish with the toasted sesame oil. Taste and add a squeeze of lemon if you like a bright note.

Why this helps your bones and daily energy

Tofu made with calcium sulfate provides calcium in each serving, and the protein supports muscle repair after strength sessions. Leafy greens contribute vitamin K, which helps guide calcium into bone tissue, and magnesium, which supports the mineral matrix and muscle function. Sesame seeds add extra calcium and healthy fats that make the meal satisfying. The gentle spice from ginger can aid digestion, and turmeric offers a warm color and a small antioxidant boost. Together these ingredients create a steady meal that keeps energy even through the morning or evening.

Safe prep and easy variations

If you prefer a softer texture, add two spoons of fortified plant milk near the end and stir until creamy. If you avoid soy, use crumbled chickpea tofu or soft scrambled eggs and add extra sesame and greens for minerals. For a higher protein option, stir in edamame or a spoon of cottage cheese at the end if you tolerate dairy. If sodium is a concern, use low sodium tamari and rinse the tofu well. To make a portable option, spoon the scramble into a whole grain wrap and fold it while still warm, then let it set for a minute so it holds together.

How to serve and store

Serve the scramble warm with a slice of whole grain toast or a bowl of brown rice. Sprinkle sesame seeds over the top just before eating for aroma and crunch. Leftovers keep well in a covered container for up to two days and reheat gently in a pan with a splash of water. The flavors deepen overnight, so this recipe works well for make ahead lunches.

Gentle coaching note

If tofu is new in your kitchen, start with a half block and notice how you feel. Check the label for calcium sulfate so you know you are getting the benefit. Meals like this, repeated during the week, add small deposits to your bone bank while keeping your routine simple.

Tahini Chickpea Bowl with Roasted Broccoli and Lemon

This warm bowl is creamy, bright, and built from pantry staples. Tahini provides calcium in a plant form. Chickpeas add protein and fiber that keep energy steady. Broccoli brings vitamin K and vitamin C. A touch of lemon lifts the flavors so the dish tastes fresh even on busy nights.

Ingredients and prep in plain words

Open a can of chickpeas, drain, and rinse them. Cut a medium head of broccoli into bite size florets and slice the stalk thinly so nothing is wasted. Keep a small red onion or a shallot, a clove of garlic, and a lemon. Stir tahini with warm water to loosen it and keep extra virgin olive oil, sea salt, and black pepper nearby. If you enjoy spice, keep a pinch of chili flakes. Have a cup of cooked brown rice or quinoa ready, or plan to toast a slice of whole grain bread to serve alongside.

Method explained step by step in sentences

Heat the oven to a moderate temperature and spread the broccoli on a tray. Drizzle with a little olive oil, add a pinch of salt, and roast until the edges turn lightly browned and the stems are tender. While the broccoli cooks, warm a pan and soften the sliced onion in a spoon of olive oil with a small pinch of salt. Add the garlic and stir briefly so the aroma rises without browning. Tip in the chickpeas with a splash of water and let them become glossy and warm. In a small bowl whisk tahini with warm water and a squeeze of lemon until it turns smooth and pourable. Add a pinch of salt and a grind of pepper. When the broccoli is ready, combine it with the chickpeas in the pan and pour the tahini sauce over the mixture. Stir gently over low heat until the sauce coats everything and turns creamy. Add more warm water if it becomes too thick. Finish with lemon zest and a few drops of juice to taste.

Why this helps your bones and daily energy

Tahini made from sesame seeds delivers calcium and healthy fats that slow digestion and make meals satisfying. Chickpeas supply protein to support muscle repair and give a steady release of energy. Broccoli adds vitamin K, which helps direct calcium into bone, and vitamin C, which supports collagen formation. The fiber in chickpeas and whole grains supports gut health, which may help with nutrient absorption. Olive oil adds a smooth mouthfeel and supports heart health.

Safe prep and easy variations

If you prefer softer textures, cook the broccoli a little longer and mash some chickpeas with the back of a spoon so the sauce becomes thicker and creamier. If sodium is a concern, season with lemon and herbs instead of extra salt. If you need more protein, stir in a spoon of Greek yogurt at the end off the heat, or toss in cubes of calcium set tofu. If you avoid sesame, blend soaked cashews with warm water and lemon to replace tahini, or use sunflower seed butter. For a grain free option, serve the bowl on a bed of wilted greens.

How to serve and store

Serve the bowl over warm brown rice or quinoa, or spoon it beside toasted whole grain bread. Scatter a few extra sesame seeds or chopped parsley on top if you like a fresh note. Leftovers keep well in a covered container for two days and reheat gently with a splash of water to loosen the sauce. The flavors settle and become rounder by the next day, making this a good choice for packed lunches.

Gentle coaching note

Bowls like this are easy to repeat on busy weeks. Keep a jar of tahini in the cupboard and a bag of frozen broccoli as a backup. With chickpeas on your shelf you can build a calcium and protein rich meal in less time than it takes to order delivery.

Baked Salmon Oat Cakes with Lemon Yogurt Sauce

These tender cakes use canned salmon with the soft bones included, which adds calcium and vitamin D along with high quality protein. Oats make the texture moist and hold the mixture together without heavy breadcrumbs. Baking keeps the crust crisp and the inside soft. A quick lemon yogurt sauce adds brightness and extra protein.

Ingredients and prep in plain words

Open one large can of salmon packed in water, including the soft bones. Drain well. Finely chop a small onion and a stalk of celery. Crack two eggs into a bowl and beat them lightly with a fork. Measure a cup of quick oats or rolled oats pulsed a few times in a blender, a spoon of Dijon mustard, a squeeze of lemon juice, a spoon of chopped parsley or dill, and a pinch of salt and pepper. For the sauce, stir plain Greek yogurt with lemon zest, a squeeze of juice, and a little olive oil. Keep olive oil spray or a brush ready for the tray.

Method explained step by step in sentences

Heat the oven to a moderate temperature and line a tray with baking paper. Brush or spray the paper lightly with olive oil. Tip the salmon into a large bowl and break it into flakes with a fork, letting the soft bones crumble into the mixture. Add the onion, celery, mustard, parsley, oats, beaten eggs, lemon juice, salt, and pepper. Stir gently until everything holds together. If the mix looks wet, add a spoon or two more oats and wait a minute so they absorb moisture. With damp hands form small patties about the size of your palm and place them on the tray. Brush the tops with a little olive oil. Bake until the cakes are firm and golden at the edges, turning them once halfway so both sides crisp. While they bake, mix the yogurt sauce and taste for lemon and salt. Let the cakes rest for a few minutes after baking so they set, then serve warm with the sauce.

Why this helps your bones and daily energy

Canned salmon with bones provides calcium in a form your body can use and natural vitamin D that helps you absorb calcium. The protein in salmon and yogurt supports muscle repair, which is key when you are training with weights or bands. Oats add soluble fiber that steadies blood sugar and small amounts of magnesium and phosphorus, both part of the bone matrix. Herbs and lemon bring flavor without excess salt.

Safe prep and easy variations

If you prefer dairy free, use a soy or coconut yogurt for the sauce or replace it with tahini whisked with lemon and water. If sodium is a concern, choose low sodium canned salmon and season the mixture with lemon and herbs rather than extra salt. For a softer texture, bake the patties a little less so the center stays tender. If you want more crunch, brush the tops lightly with olive oil just before the final minutes of baking. To make them gluten free, confirm the oats are certified gluten free.

How to serve and store

Serve the cakes with a side of leafy greens dressed with olive oil and lemon, or place them on whole grain buns with lettuce for a simple sandwich. They pack well for lunches. Store leftovers in a covered container in the fridge for up to two days and reheat in a hot oven for a few minutes so the edges crisp again.

Gentle coaching note

Keeping a can of salmon and a bag of oats in the pantry means you can make a bone friendly dinner any time. These cakes also freeze well after baking. Reheat directly from frozen in a warm oven so dinner is ready when you come home from training.

Spinach Mushroom Ricotta Frittata (Oven Baked)

This frittata is soft, savory, and rich in protein and calcium. Baking in the oven keeps the texture tender and removes the need to flip, which makes it friendly for days when you want a calm kitchen. It works for breakfast, lunch, or a light dinner and tastes good warm or at room temperature.

Ingredients and prep in plain words

Crack six large eggs into a bowl. In another bowl stir half a cup of ricotta and half a cup of plain Greek yogurt until smooth. Rinse a large handful of baby spinach and slice a cup of mushrooms. Grate a small piece of hard cheese if you enjoy it, such as Parmesan or a mild cheddar, about a quarter cup. Chop a small onion. Keep olive oil, salt, and black pepper nearby. If you like herbs, prepare chopped parsley or chives. Heat the oven and place a lightly oiled ovenproof pan or pie dish on the counter.

Method explained step by step in sentences

Warm a pan over medium heat with a spoon of olive oil. Soften the chopped onion with a small pinch of salt until it turns translucent. Add the sliced mushrooms and cook until they release their juices and become golden at the edges. Add the spinach and stir until it wilts and turns glossy. Turn off the heat and let the vegetables cool for a minute. In the bowl with eggs, whisk until the yolks and whites combine. Stir in the ricotta and yogurt mixture until the batter looks smooth. Add a pinch of salt and a grind of pepper. Fold the vegetables into the egg mixture and pour it into the oiled ovenproof dish. Sprinkle the grated cheese on top if using. Bake until the center is just set and a knife inserted near the middle comes out clean. Let the frittata rest for five minutes so it slices neatly.

Why this helps your bones and daily energy

Eggs and yogurt supply complete protein that supports muscle repair after strength work. Ricotta and a small amount of hard cheese add calcium. Spinach brings vitamin K and magnesium, which support bone metabolism, even though its calcium is less absorbable; it still contributes micronutrients and flavor. Mushrooms provide texture and small amounts of vitamin D when exposed to light. The result is a gentle, satisfying meal that keeps you steady for hours.

Safe prep and easy variations

If you avoid dairy, replace ricotta and yogurt with a silky blend of soft tofu and a spoon of olive oil, then season with lemon to lift the flavor. If sodium is a concern, skip the hard cheese and season with herbs and pepper. For extra protein, add a small handful of cottage cheese to the mixture if you tolerate dairy. If the top browns too quickly, cover loosely with foil for the last minutes. To make portions easy to handle, bake the mixture in a lined muffin tray and reduce the baking time.

How to serve and store

Serve slices with a side of ripe tomatoes or a simple salad dressed with olive oil and lemon. For a heartier meal add a slice of whole grain bread. Leftovers keep well in the fridge for up to two days and reheat gently or taste good cold. The texture stays moist, which helps on days when chewing is tiring.

Gentle coaching note

Baked egg dishes are an easy way to place protein and calcium at the center of a meal without long prep. Keep a tub of ricotta or a block of soft tofu in the fridge and a bag of spinach in the freezer so this recipe is always within reach.

Cottage Cheese Oat Pancakes with Blueberries

These soft pancakes are high in protein and calcium, gentle on digestion, and quick to make. Oats add fiber and magnesium. Blueberries bring vitamin C and natural sweetness. The batter blends smooth, so cooking is calm and the texture stays tender.

Ingredients and prep in plain words

Measure one cup of cottage cheese and one cup of rolled oats. Crack two large eggs. Add half a cup of milk or fortified soy milk. Keep a teaspoon of baking powder, a pinch of salt, and half a teaspoon of vanilla if you enjoy it. Rinse a cup of fresh or frozen blueberries. Have a little butter or olive oil for the pan and some plain yogurt for serving if you like.

Method explained step by step in sentences

Place the cottage cheese, oats, eggs, milk, baking powder, salt, and vanilla into a blender. Blend until the mixture turns smooth and slightly thick. Let it rest for a few minutes so the oats hydrate and the batter firms a little. Warm a nonstick pan over medium heat and brush it lightly with butter or oil. Pour small circles of batter into the pan. Drop a few blueberries on each pancake and press them gently so they sink in. Cook until small bubbles appear at the surface and the edges look set, then flip with a thin spatula and cook the second side until golden. Adjust the heat so the pancakes cook through without burning. Repeat with the remaining batter, brushing the pan lightly between batches.

Why this helps your bones and daily energy

Cottage cheese brings a reliable dose of calcium and complete protein. Eggs add more protein and support muscle repair after strength training. Oats provide fiber and magnesium, which supports the bone mineral matrix and muscle function. Fortified soy milk increases calcium and vitamin D, which helps your body absorb calcium from the meal. Blueberries add vitamin C that supports collagen formation. Together these nutrients build a steady breakfast or recovery snack.

Safe prep and easy variations

If you avoid dairy, use a thick soy yogurt or a smooth tofu blend in place of cottage cheese and choose fortified soy or almond milk for the liquid. If sodium is a concern, choose low sodium cottage cheese and skip extra salt. For a softer texture, blend longer and cook the pancakes smaller so they flip easily. If you need more energy after training, serve with a spoon of nut butter or a drizzle of warm tahini mixed with a little honey or maple.

How to serve and store

Serve warm with a spoon of yogurt or a squeeze of lemon and a few extra berries. These pancakes keep well in the fridge for two days and reheat in a dry pan or toaster on low. They also freeze well. Stack cooled pancakes between small squares of baking paper and store in a freezer bag. Reheat from frozen in a warm pan for a quick, bone friendly breakfast.

Gentle coaching note

Batch cooking helps on busy weeks. Make a double recipe on a calm day and freeze portions. Having a ready protein and calcium source in the morning sets the tone for steady energy and better training later in the day.

White Bean, Kale, and Parmesan Rind Soup

This is a calm, comforting soup that comes together with pantry staples. White beans bring protein and fiber. Kale adds vitamin K and magnesium. A small piece of Parmesan rind melts slowly and gives calcium and deep flavor. The broth stays clear and gentle, which makes it friendly for days when you want something warm but not heavy.

Ingredients and prep in plain words

Open two cans of white beans and rinse them. Rinse a large bunch of kale, strip the leaves, and slice them thinly. Keep one small onion, one carrot, and one stalk of celery. Peel a clove of garlic. Find a small piece of Parmesan rind if you have it. If you avoid dairy, you can skip the rind and finish with lemon and olive oil. Measure six cups of low sodium vegetable or chicken broth, two spoons of olive oil, a bay leaf, and a pinch of chili flakes if you like gentle heat. Keep black pepper and salt nearby.

Method explained step by step in sentences

Warm a pot over medium heat and add the olive oil. Soften the chopped onion, carrot, and celery with a pinch of salt until they turn glossy. Add the sliced garlic and stir for a minute so the aroma rises. Tip in the beans and stir so they shine with oil. Pour in the broth and add the bay leaf and the Parmesan rind. Bring the pot to a gentle simmer and cook for about fifteen minutes so the flavors blend. Mash a few beans against the side of the pot to thicken the soup slightly. Add the sliced kale and simmer for another five to seven minutes until the greens are tender but still bright. Remove the bay leaf and the rind. Taste and adjust with salt and black pepper. If you skipped the rind, finish with a squeeze of lemon and a drizzle of olive oil for depth.

Why this helps your bones and daily energy

White beans provide plant protein that supports muscle repair. They also offer small amounts of calcium and magnesium that add up over the week. Kale delivers vitamin K, which helps guide calcium into bone tissue, and magnesium, which supports the mineral matrix. The Parmesan rind contributes calcium and flavor without needing a large amount of cheese. A clear broth keeps the meal light yet steady so energy does not spike and crash.

Safe prep and easy variations

If you prefer a softer texture, cook the soup a little longer and mash more beans into the broth. If you want extra protein, stir in shredded chicken breast near the end or add cubes of calcium set tofu. If sodium is a concern, use low sodium broth and season with herbs, lemon, and black pepper. If you enjoy grains, add a handful of small pasta or cooked farro to the bowls before ladling the soup so the texture stays pleasant.

How to serve and store

Serve the soup hot with a slice of whole grain bread or a spoon of brown rice in the bowl. A sprinkle of chopped parsley adds freshness. Leftovers keep well for three days in the fridge and reheat gently. The soup also freezes well. Cool it first, portion into containers, and leave space at the top for expansion. Reheat from thawed over low heat and adjust with a splash of water if it has thickened.

Gentle coaching note

Soups like this are easy to repeat and kind to your schedule. Keep a jar of Parmesan rinds in the freezer and a couple of cans of beans in the cupboard. With greens and broth on hand, you have a warm, bone friendly meal ready whenever you need it.

Yogurt-Lemon Chicken Thighs with Sesame Broccoli

This tray bake is simple, juicy, and built to support bone health. A yogurt and lemon marinade keeps the chicken tender and adds calcium and protein. Broccoli brings vitamin K and fiber. Sesame finishes the vegetables with a nutty scent and a little extra calcium.

Ingredients and prep in plain words

Trim eight small boneless, skinless chicken thighs. In a bowl mix one cup of plain Greek yogurt, the zest and juice of one lemon, two cloves of garlic finely grated, a spoon of olive oil, a teaspoon of dried oregano, a pinch of salt, and black pepper. Cut one large head of broccoli into bite size pieces. Have a spoon of sesame seeds and a teaspoon of toasted sesame oil ready. If you like heat, keep a pinch of chili flakes. Line a large baking tray with paper and heat the oven to a moderate temperature.

Method explained step by step in sentences

Coat the chicken thighs in the yogurt mixture and let them rest while you prepare the broccoli. Spread the broccoli on the lined tray and drizzle with a little olive oil and a small pinch of salt. Push the broccoli to one side and place the marinated chicken on the other side, letting extra marinade cling to each piece. Bake until the chicken is cooked through and the broccoli edges are browned, turning the broccoli once so it roasts evenly. When the tray comes out, scatter sesame seeds over the hot broccoli and drizzle the sesame oil so the aroma rises. Let the chicken rest for a few minutes, then spoon any juices from the tray over the pieces.

Why this helps your bones and daily energy

Greek yogurt contributes calcium and complete protein, both essential for bone and muscle. Chicken thighs provide iron and additional protein for recovery after training. Broccoli adds vitamin K, which helps guide calcium into bone tissue, plus vitamin C for collagen support. Sesame seeds add a small but meaningful boost of calcium and healthy fats that make the meal satisfying without heaviness.

Safe prep and easy variations

If you avoid dairy, marinate the chicken in olive oil, lemon, garlic, and a spoon of tahini for creaminess, then thin with warm water. If sodium is a concern, season lightly and use extra lemon and herbs for brightness. For a softer vegetable texture, steam the broccoli for two minutes before roasting so it turns tender more quickly. You can swap broccoli for bok choy or kale; add greens near the end so they wilt without burning. If you prefer white meat, use chicken breasts cut in half and bake for a shorter time so they stay juicy.

How to serve and store

Serve with brown rice, quinoa, or roasted potatoes. Spoon the pan juices over the grains so nothing is lost. Leftovers keep well in a covered container for two days and reheat gently. The yogurt marinade keeps the chicken moist even after chilling.

Gentle coaching note

Tray bakes reduce effort on busy nights. Pairing a calcium rich marinade with a vitamin K rich vegetable turns a simple dinner into a steady deposit for bone health. Write this recipe on your weekly plan and repeat it whenever training runs late.

Silken Tofu Berry Smoothie (Dairy Free, Calcium and Protein)

This creamy smoothie is a quick option for busy mornings or a gentle recovery snack after training. It uses fortified soy milk and silken tofu for calcium and protein without dairy. Berries add vitamin C for collagen support, and chia seeds contribute fiber and extra calcium.

Ingredients and prep in plain words

Measure one cup of chilled fortified soy milk. Open a small pack of silken tofu and measure half a cup. Rinse one cup of mixed berries, fresh or frozen. Measure one tablespoon of chia seeds and one teaspoon of maple syrup or honey if you enjoy a touch of sweetness. Add a small squeeze of lemon for brightness and a few ice cubes if you like a colder drink.

Method explained step by step in sentences

Place the soy milk, silken tofu, berries, chia seeds, lemon, and sweetener in a blender. Blend on high until the mixture turns completely smooth and lightly thick. If the smoothie looks too thick, add a splash of soy milk and blend again. If it looks thin, add a few more berries or a few extra cubes of tofu and blend once more. Taste and adjust the lemon or sweetness to your preference. Pour into a glass and let it sit for two minutes so the chia seeds begin to thicken the texture slightly.

Why this helps your bones and daily energy

Fortified soy milk provides calcium and vitamin D that help your body absorb calcium efficiently. Silken tofu adds complete plant protein and extra calcium when the tofu is set with calcium salts. Berries offer vitamin C for collagen formation and antioxidants that support recovery. Chia seeds contribute calcium, fiber, and healthy fats that make the smoothie satisfying and steady in energy.

Safe prep and easy variations

If you prefer a richer texture, add a spoon of almond butter. If you need to avoid soy, use calcium fortified almond milk and replace tofu with a scoop of plain whey or a neutral plant protein. If you want more energy for long walks, add half a banana or a spoon of rolled oats before blending. If you like greens, add a small handful of baby spinach; the color changes but the flavor stays mild.

How to serve and store

Drink the smoothie soon after blending for the best texture. If you need to carry it, pour it into an insulated bottle and keep it cold. Shake before drinking because chia can thicken on standing. For batch prep, blend the berries and tofu without the chia, freeze in portions, then add soy milk and chia when you are ready to drink so the texture stays fresh.

Gentle coaching note

Smoothies like this are helpful on days when appetite is low. They deliver calcium and protein in a form that is easy to sip and kind to your schedule, keeping your training and recovery on track.

Ricotta Lemon Stuffed Sweet Potatoes with Garlicky Kale

This cozy dish brings together soft sweet potatoes, a bright ricotta filling, and a tangle of warm kale. It is gentle to chew, easy to assemble, and rich in protein, calcium, vitamin K, and magnesium. The flavors are clean and comforting, which makes it a steady weeknight meal.

Ingredients and prep in plain words

Choose two medium sweet potatoes. Rinse them and pierce the skins with a fork. In a bowl stir one cup of ricotta with the zest of half a lemon, a squeeze of lemon juice, a pinch of salt, and black pepper. Grate a small clove of garlic and chop a handful of parsley. Rinse a large bunch of kale, strip the leaves from the stems, and slice them thinly. Keep a tablespoon of olive oil, a teaspoon of butter or more olive oil, and a spoon of grated hard cheese if you enjoy it. Have chili flakes if you like gentle heat.

Method explained step by step in sentences

Heat the oven to a moderate temperature. Rub the sweet potatoes lightly with olive oil and place them on a small tray. Bake until a knife slips through the centers without resistance. While they cook, warm a wide pan over medium heat with a spoon of olive oil. Add the grated garlic and let it sizzle for a few seconds without browning. Pile the sliced kale into the pan with a small pinch of salt and stir until it wilts and turns glossy. Add a splash of water if the pan looks dry. When the kale is tender, turn off the heat and keep it warm. In a bowl, taste the ricotta mixture and adjust with a little more lemon or salt if needed. When the sweet potatoes are ready, let them cool for a minute so steam escapes. Split each potato lengthwise and gently press the ends to open the centers. Use a fork to fluff the flesh and stir in a small knob of butter or a drizzle of olive oil with a pinch of salt. Spoon half of the lemon ricotta into each potato and let the warmth soften it. Top with a mound of garlicky kale. Finish with chopped parsley, a few chili flakes if you like, and a light sprinkle of grated hard cheese for aroma.

Why this helps your bones and daily energy

Ricotta provides calcium and high quality protein that support bone mineralization and muscle repair, especially useful on training days. Kale contributes vitamin K, which helps guide calcium into bone tissue, and magnesium, which supports the mineral matrix and muscle function. Sweet potatoes add potassium and steady carbohydrates that keep energy even. Olive oil gives a smooth mouthfeel and supports heart health, making the dish satisfying without heaviness.

Safe prep and easy variations

If you avoid dairy, replace ricotta with a blend of silken tofu, lemon juice, a pinch of salt, and a spoon of olive oil; blitz until creamy. If sodium is a concern, season more with lemon zest and herbs and use a light hand with cheese. For extra protein, stir a spoon of cottage cheese into the ricotta or add a handful of white beans to the kale in the pan. If chewing is difficult, mash the sweet potato flesh fully with the ricotta and spoon the kale very finely sliced over the top for a softer texture. To add crunch, toast a spoon of pumpkin seeds in a dry pan and scatter them just before serving; they add magnesium and a nutty note.

How to serve and store

Serve each stuffed potato as a full meal or pair with a small side salad dressed with olive oil and lemon. The dish packs well for lunch. Let the potatoes cool, close them gently, and store in a covered container for up to two days. Reheat in a warm oven until hot through or in a microwave at low power so the filling warms without drying out.

Gentle coaching note

Baking a few sweet potatoes at once turns future meals into five minute assemblies. Keep lemon ricotta ready in the fridge and a bag of kale washed and sliced. On busy nights you will have a calcium and vitamin K rich dinner on the table with little effort.

Kefir Overnight Oats with Chia and Almonds

This no-cook breakfast sits in the fridge while you sleep and greets you with calm energy in the morning. Kefir provides calcium, protein, and live cultures that support digestion. Oats and chia bring fiber and magnesium. Almonds add crunch and extra calcium. The texture is creamy and gentle, and the flavor can be brightened with lemon and fruit.

Ingredients and prep in plain words

Measure half a cup of rolled oats and place them in a jar or small bowl. Pour in three quarters of a cup of plain kefir. Stir in a tablespoon of chia seeds and a teaspoon of honey or maple if you like mild sweetness. Add a small squeeze of lemon and a pinch of zest for freshness. Chop a small handful of almonds. Rinse half a cup of fresh fruit such as sliced strawberries, blueberries, or diced pear. Keep a pinch of cinnamon nearby if you enjoy warm notes.

Method explained step by step in sentences

Stir the oats, kefir, chia, lemon, and sweetener in the jar until everything is wet and evenly mixed. Cover and place in the fridge for at least four hours, ideally overnight, so the oats soften and the chia thickens the mixture. In the morning, open the jar and stir once more to loosen the texture. If it looks too thick, add a splash of kefir or milk and stir again. If it looks thin, add a spoon of yogurt or a few extra oats and let it sit for five minutes. Fold in most of the fruit and almonds, saving a little for the top. Dust with a pinch of cinnamon if you like and finish with the remaining fruit and nuts so the first spoonful tastes bright and crisp.

Why this helps your bones and daily energy

Kefir delivers calcium and complete protein in a form that many people find easy to digest. Its live cultures can support a healthy gut environment, which may help with nutrient absorption. Oats provide soluble fiber and magnesium that support muscle and bone function. Chia seeds contribute calcium and healthy fats that slow digestion for even energy. Almonds add more calcium and magnesium in a crunchy form that feels satisfying. Fruit brings vitamin C to support collagen formation, pairing well with calcium-rich dairy.

Safe prep and easy variations

If you avoid dairy, use calcium-fortified soy or almond milk with a spoon of soy yogurt in place of kefir. If you need lower sugar, skip sweeteners and rely on fruit and cinnamon for flavor. If you prefer a smoother texture, pulse the oats briefly in a blender before mixing so they soften more. If nuts are not suitable, use pumpkin seeds for crunch and extra magnesium. For added protein, stir in a spoon of cottage cheese or a scoop of plain whey or plant protein just before eating.

How to serve and store

Eat directly from the jar for a quick breakfast or spoon into a bowl and add extra fruit if you have time. This mixture keeps for two days in the fridge, which makes it useful for batch prep. If you plan to store it longer than one night, add the chopped almonds just before serving so they stay crisp.

Gentle coaching note

Place two jars in the fridge on calm evenings so your future self has a ready, calcium-rich breakfast. Small habits like this support steady training and clearer mornings without extra effort.

Orange Sesame Tofu with Bok Choy (Calcium Set, One Pan)

This quick stir-fry is bright, tender, and built to support bones. Calcium-set tofu supplies absorbable calcium and protein, while bok choy adds vitamin K and vitamin C. A light orange-sesame sauce coats everything without heaviness. The textures are soft and the flavors are fresh, so it works on busy nights or after training.

Ingredients and prep in plain words

Choose a firm block of tofu that lists calcium sulfate on the label. Press it briefly between towels and cut into bite-size cubes. Rinse two small heads of bok choy and slice them, keeping stems and leaves separate. Peel a small clove of garlic and grate a thumb of fresh ginger. In a cup, stir the zest of half an orange with its juice, a spoon of low-sodium soy sauce or tamari, a teaspoon of honey or maple, a teaspoon of rice vinegar, and half a teaspoon of toasted sesame oil. In another cup, mix half a teaspoon of cornstarch with two spoons of cold water. Keep a spoon of sesame seeds and a little neutral oil for the pan.

Method explained step by step in sentences

Warm a wide nonstick pan over medium heat with a thin film of oil. Add the tofu cubes in a single layer and let them take on light color on one side before turning them gently so the edges become golden. Slide the tofu to the edge of the pan. Add a few drops of oil to the center and stir the grated ginger and garlic for thirty seconds so the aroma rises without browning. Tip in the bok choy stems and cook until they begin to soften and look glossy. Add the leaves and stir until they wilt. Pour in the orange mixture and let it bubble for a moment. Stir the cornstarch slurry and add it to the pan. Toss gently until the sauce turns clear and silkier and coats the tofu and greens. Sprinkle sesame seeds over the top and turn off the heat. Taste and add a squeeze more orange or a splash of soy if needed.

Why this helps your bones and daily energy

Calcium-set tofu delivers calcium in each portion and provides complete plant protein to support muscle repair. Bok choy contributes vitamin K, which helps direct calcium into bone tissue, and vitamin C, which supports collagen formation. Sesame seeds add a small boost of calcium and healthy fats that make the dish satisfying. The light sauce keeps flavors bright without excess sodium or sugar, which helps you feel steady after eating.

Safe prep and easy variations

If you need softer textures, cook the bok choy a minute longer and cut tofu into smaller cubes so each bite is tender. If soy is not suitable, replace tofu with cooked chicken breast pieces and add a spoon of tahini to the sauce for creaminess. If you prefer no cornstarch, reduce the sauce a bit longer until it naturally thickens. For extra protein, toss in a handful of edamame or cashews near the end. If sodium is a concern, use low-sodium tamari and rely on orange zest and ginger for bright flavor.

How to serve and store

Serve over warm brown rice or quinoa, or spoon it beside cauliflower rice for a lighter plate. Leftovers keep well in a covered container for up to two days and reheat gently with a splash of water to loosen the sauce. The citrus aroma remains fresh on day two, making this a good make-ahead lunch.

Gentle coaching note

Keep a block of calcium-set tofu and a couple of bok choy in your fridge. With an orange and a spoon of sesame seeds, you can put a calcium and vitamin K rich dinner on the table in under twenty minutes.

No Bake Almond Tahini Calcium Bites (Travel Friendly Snack)

These small bites travel well, keep in the fridge for days, and give a calm, steady lift between meals. Tahini supplies calcium in a plant form. Almonds add more calcium and magnesium. Oats bring fiber that makes the snack satisfying without heaviness. A touch of citrus keeps the flavor bright so one or two pieces feel enough.

Ingredients and prep in plain words

Spoon half a cup of tahini into a bowl and stir it until smooth. Finely chop half a cup of roasted almonds, or pulse them in a blender until they look like coarse crumbs. Measure three quarters of a cup of quick oats. Grate the zest of half an orange or lemon and squeeze a little juice. Add two tablespoons of honey or maple syrup, a pinch of salt, and half a teaspoon of vanilla if you enjoy it. Keep two tablespoons of finely chopped dried apricots or raisins if you like small sweet pops, and a spoon of sesame seeds for rolling.

Method explained step by step in sentences

Stir the tahini, honey, citrus zest, and a small squeeze of juice in the bowl until the mixture loosens and turns glossy. Tip in the chopped almonds and oats and fold with a spoon until everything is evenly coated. If using dried fruit, add it now and mix again. Let the bowl rest for five minutes so the oats absorb moisture. If the mixture looks too soft to shape, add a little more oats. If it looks dry, add a teaspoon of orange juice. Rub a little tahini or water on your palms and roll small portions into bite size balls. Scatter sesame seeds on a plate and roll each ball lightly so a thin coat clings to the surface. Place the bites on a small tray and refrigerate for at least twenty minutes so they set and hold together.

Why this helps your bones and daily energy

Tahini made from sesame seeds provides calcium and healthy fats that slow digestion and keep energy even. Almonds add more calcium and magnesium and contribute a pleasant crunch. Oats bring fiber and small amounts of minerals that support the bone matrix. A gentle dose of natural sugars from honey and dried fruit pairs with fats and fiber so the release of energy is steady rather than sharp. These bites help you arrive at training or travel connections with a clear head.

Safe prep and easy variations

If you prefer lower sugar, reduce the honey and add a spoon of plain peanut butter for extra richness. If you need nut free, replace almonds with toasted pumpkin seeds for magnesium and a similar crunch. If you avoid gluten, choose certified gluten free oats. For a softer texture, pulse the whole mixture briefly in a blender before shaping. If you want extra protein after strength sessions, stir in a small scoop of plain whey or plant protein and adjust texture with a splash more citrus juice.

How to serve and store

Eat one or two bites with tea or after a walk. Pack them in a small box with baking paper between layers so they do not stick. They keep in the fridge for one week and freeze well for a month. Let them soften at room temperature for a few minutes before eating if frozen.

Gentle coaching note

Keeping a tray of these in the fridge reduces the chance of skipping protein and calcium between meals. They are also a friendly option before lifting grandchildren or suitcases because they steady energy without a heavy stomach.

Turkey Ricotta Meatballs in Spinach Tomato Sauce

These tender meatballs simmer in a bright tomato sauce and finish with a handful of spinach for vitamin K. Ricotta keeps the texture soft and adds calcium and protein. The dish is gentle, comforting, and easy to portion for future meals.

Ingredients and prep in plain words

Choose five hundred grams of lean ground turkey. In a bowl place half a cup of ricotta, one egg, two tablespoons of finely grated Parmesan or pecorino if you enjoy it, and one small garlic clove finely grated. Add half a cup of quick oats or fresh breadcrumbs, a pinch of salt, black pepper, and a tablespoon of chopped parsley. For the sauce, open one large can of crushed tomatoes, slice a small onion, and keep a tablespoon of olive oil. Rinse a large handful of baby spinach. Have lemon on hand to brighten the sauce.

Method explained step by step in sentences

In a large bowl mix the ricotta, egg, Parmesan, garlic, oats, salt, pepper, and parsley until smooth. Add the ground turkey and fold gently with a fork until just combined. Wet your hands and roll small meatballs about the size of a walnut. Warm a wide pan over medium heat with the olive oil. Brown the meatballs in batches until they take on light color on two sides; they do not need to cook through yet. Set them aside on a plate. In the same pan soften the sliced onion with a pinch of salt until translucent. Pour in the crushed tomatoes and bring to a gentle simmer. Return the meatballs to the pan, nestling them into the sauce. Cover and cook over low heat until the meatballs are cooked through and tender. Stir in the spinach until it wilts. Taste the sauce and brighten with a squeeze of lemon and a grind of pepper.

Why this helps your bones and daily energy

Turkey provides lean protein that supports muscle repair after training. Ricotta and a little Parmesan add calcium for bone mineralization. Spinach contributes vitamin K and magnesium that support bone metabolism. Oats in the mixture bring soft fiber and small amounts of minerals while keeping the texture moist. Olive oil supports heart health and helps fat-soluble vitamins do their work. The result is a steady meal that keeps energy even.

Safe prep and easy variations

If you avoid dairy, replace ricotta with soft tofu blended with a teaspoon of olive oil and a squeeze of lemon, and skip Parmesan. If sodium is a concern, season lightly and rely on lemon, garlic, and fresh herbs for flavor. For extra protein, stir a spoon of cottage cheese into a portion after cooking if you tolerate dairy. If you need a softer texture, simmer the meatballs a few minutes longer so they become very tender and chop the spinach finely before adding it. If you prefer beef or chicken, swap the turkey and keep the same method.

How to serve and store

Serve the meatballs over polenta, whole grain pasta, or a bowl of brown rice. Spoon extra sauce over the top and finish with parsley. Leftovers keep well in a covered container for three days and freeze nicely for a month. Reheat gently over low heat with a splash of water so the sauce loosens without sticking.

Gentle coaching note

Batch cooking meatballs gives you ready protein and calcium for busy days. Freeze portions of four meatballs with sauce so a balanced meal is always within reach after training or travel.

Lemon Tahini Lentil Pilaf with Leafy Greens

This one-pan pilaf is comforting and bright. Lentils bring steady protein and minerals. A lemon tahini finish adds plant calcium and a smooth, savory note. Leafy greens fold in at the end for vitamin K and magnesium. The texture stays soft and moist, which makes it friendly on days when you want a gentle meal.

Ingredients and prep in plain words

Rinse one cup of green or brown lentils. Rinse half a cup of long-grain rice or quinoa if you prefer. Slice one small onion and a clove of garlic. Rinse a large handful of chopped kale or spinach. Zest one lemon and squeeze its juice. In a cup whisk two tablespoons tahini with two tablespoons warm water and a tablespoon of lemon juice until smooth. Keep two tablespoons of olive oil, half a teaspoon of ground cumin, a pinch of salt, and black pepper. If you enjoy herbs, chop a small handful of parsley. Have low-sodium vegetable broth ready, about three cups.

Method explained step by step in sentences

Warm a wide pot over medium heat and add the olive oil. Soften the sliced onion with a small pinch of salt until it turns glossy. Add the garlic and ground cumin and stir for thirty seconds so the aroma rises. Tip in the rinsed lentils and rice and stir so the grains shine with oil. Pour in the broth and bring to a gentle simmer. Cover and cook until the lentils are tender and the rice is soft, adding a splash of hot water if the pot looks dry. When the grains are almost done, fold in the chopped greens and cook for a few minutes until they wilt and turn tender. Turn off the heat. Stir the lemon zest through the pilaf. Whisk the tahini mixture again and drizzle it over the pot. Fold gently so some sauce clings to the grains and some stays in soft ribbons. Taste and adjust with more lemon, salt, or pepper.

Why this helps your bones and daily energy

Lentils provide plant protein and minerals such as magnesium and phosphorus that support the bone matrix. The lemon-tahini sauce delivers calcium in a plant form and healthy fats that create a steady release of energy. Leafy greens contribute vitamin K, which helps direct calcium into bone tissue, and magnesium, which supports muscle function. The mix of protein, complex carbohydrates, and fats keeps you full and ready for training or travel.

Safe prep and easy variations

If you prefer softer textures, use red lentils and cook a little longer with extra broth to create a spoonable stew. If you avoid sesame, replace tahini with plain Greek yogurt thinned with lemon, or with blended cashews for a dairy free option. If sodium is a concern, use water instead of broth and season with lemon, cumin, and parsley. For extra protein, fold in cubes of calcium-set tofu at the end or top portions with a spoon of cottage cheese if you tolerate dairy. If rice is not your choice, swap in quinoa and reduce liquid slightly because quinoa cooks faster.

How to serve and store

Serve warm in bowls with a squeeze of lemon and a sprinkle of parsley. A few toasted pumpkin seeds on top add crunch and extra magnesium. This pilaf keeps well for three days in the fridge. Reheat gently with a splash of water so the grains loosen and the tahini stays creamy. It also packs well for lunches and tastes good at room temperature.

Gentle coaching note

Cook a double batch on calm days and portion it into small containers. Having a calcium-rich, protein steady base ready makes it easier to keep training, posture practice, and daily walks consistent throughout a busy week.

Exercise 1

360° Rib Breathing in Tall Sit (Safe Spine Setup)

Goal in plain words

Teach your ribs to expand softly in all directions so your spine can stay long and relaxed during daily moves, lifts, and walks. This calms the nervous system and supports posture without stiffening the back.

Equipment

A sturdy chair without wheels, flat shoes or bare feet.

Starting position

Sit toward the front of the chair. Place both feet flat, hip-width apart. Stack ribs over pelvis. Let your shoulders rest wide and your chin slightly tucked so the back of the neck feels long. Place both hands around your lower ribs with thumbs at the back and fingers at the sides, forming a gentle "belt" with your hands.

How to do it (step by step)

1. Soften your belly. Imagine your torso is a quiet cylinder.

2. Inhale through the nose for a count of three. Feel your ribs widen into your thumbs, into your fingers, and a little forward under your palms. Let the breath expand sideways and back, not up into the shoulders.

3. Pause for one calm beat without holding tension.

4. Exhale through relaxed lips for a count of four to five. Feel the ribs glide inward and down while your spine stays tall. Think of "soft corset" rather than hard bracing.

5. Repeat smooth breaths, keeping the jaw unclenched and the chest from lifting.

Dosage for beginners

Five to eight slow breaths, two to three sets per day. Use it as the first minute of every workout and before lifts, carries, or step-ups.

Progression over weeks

• Place one hand on the lower ribs and the other on the belly to feel gentle abdominal support at the end of the exhale.

• Practice in standing against a wall with head and upper back lightly touching while the ribs stay stacked.

- Use the same breath during chair sit-to-stands and hip hinges (exhale on effort).

Common mistakes to avoid
Shrugging the shoulders, flaring the ribs upward, holding the breath, pushing the belly hard forward, or slumping on the chair. If the neck tightens, reset your chin to a gentle, long position.

Everyday carryover
Use this breath when standing from a chair, lifting a light bag close to your body, stepping off a curb, or picking up your grandchild. The long exhale during effort helps you move with control while keeping a neutral spine.

Safety notes for osteoporosis
Stay tall, avoid rounding forward, and keep movements slow and smooth. If you feel dizziness, stop and breathe normally for a moment before resuming.

Comic style image prompt (B/W, no text)
A single older adult seated tall on a simple chair, feet flat, neutral spine, one hand at each side of the lower ribs. Black-and-white comic illustration on a light background. Soft shading indicates 360-degree rib expansion at the sides and back. No words, letters, or

captions. Frame is mid-torso to head, calm facial expression, relaxed shoulders, clean minimal setting.

Exercise 2

Wall Tall Stand and Head Reach

Purpose in plain words
This practice teaches you to stand tall with a long neutral spine while the ribs rest quietly over the pelvis. It builds an easy sense of alignment without stiffness and prepares the body for safer walking, lifting, and balance work.

Equipment
Use a smooth wall and wear stable shoes or go barefoot.

Starting position
Stand a small step away from the wall so your pelvis and the upper back can touch lightly. Keep the knees soft. Let the shoulders rest wide. Keep the chin slightly tucked so the back of the neck feels long. Place your feet about hip width and feel equal pressure under heel, big toe base, and little toe base.

How to do it in calm steps
Breathe in through the nose and allow the ribs to widen gently to the sides and a little toward the back. As you breathe out, let the rib cage settle over the

pelvis without lifting the chest or arching the low back. Keep your gaze level with the horizon. Imagine the crown of your head reaching upward as if a thread were guiding you taller. Stay for two or three slow breaths. Now float the back of the head a finger width away from the wall while keeping the neck long and the chin easy. Hold this light reach for one or two seconds, then return the head to the wall softly. Continue to alternate gentle head reach and soft return while the rest of the body remains quiet and tall.

Dose for beginners
Practice eight to ten calm breaths in total. Repeat once or twice during the day. This makes an excellent first minute of any session before strength or balance exercises.

Progress over the weeks
Gradually increase the time you hold the tall position to three or four breaths at a time. Move the heels a little farther from the wall and keep the same alignment. When this feels natural, repeat the exercise away from the wall while standing near a sturdy surface for safety.

Common mistakes and how to correct them
Avoid pushing the head hard into the wall. Avoid

lifting the chest during inhalation. Avoid pulling the shoulders toward the ears. Avoid arching the low back. If any of these appear, reset your stance, breathe out gently, and imagine the ribs sliding back over the pelvis.

Carryover to daily life
Use the same tall feeling while waiting in line, washing dishes, standing at a counter, or riding an elevator. The long spine and quiet ribs distribute load across the back and make you feel steadier.

Safety notes for osteoporosis
Keep movements slow and controlled. Do not force the chin downward. If you feel lightheaded, stop, breathe normally, and resume only when you feel steady.

Exercise 3

Hip Hinge to Wall Tap

Purpose in plain words
Learn to bend from the hips while keeping a long neutral spine. The pelvis travels back toward the wall, the knees stay soft, and the rib cage remains quietly stacked over the pelvis. This protects the vertebrae when you reach for a bag, make a bed, or pick up a parcel.

Equipment
Use a clear wall or a closed door. Wear stable shoes or go barefoot.

Starting position
Stand facing away from the wall with your heels about twenty to thirty centimeters from the surface. Place your feet hip width and keep the toes slightly open if that feels natural. Keep your knees relaxed. Rest your hands lightly on the bony points at the front of the hips so you can feel the motion. Lengthen the back of your neck and look toward the horizon. Imagine the crown of your head growing tall.

How to do it in calm steps
Take a quiet breath in through the nose and let the ribs widen. As you breathe out, send the pelvis back as if you were about to touch the wall with your glutes. Allow the torso to tip forward while the spine stays long and the ribs remain over the pelvis. Bend the knees only as much as needed to keep comfort. When you just brush the wall with your glutes, pause for a gentle inhale without lifting the chest. Breathe out and press the feet into the floor to return to standing in one smooth motion. Finish tall without arching the low back. Repeat with the same rhythm of breath and movement.

Dose for beginners
Perform eight to ten controlled repetitions with short rests as needed. Complete two sets. Place this drill early in your session and also before household tasks that require bending.

Progress over the weeks
Move the heels a little farther from the wall to increase the travel of the pelvis. When the pattern feels steady hold a light object close to your chest such as a small backpack or a book. Over time remove the wall and practice the same hinge toward a

box or the back of a sturdy chair so the movement transfers to daily life.

Common mistakes and how to correct them
Avoid rounding the upper back, shooting the knees far forward, pushing the chin ahead of the body, or gripping the shoulders. If this happens reset the stance, think pelvis back rather than chest down, and keep the weight evenly shared between heel and forefoot. Keep the object close to the body if you choose to hold something.

Carryover to daily life
Use the hinge whenever you load a washing machine, collect a bag from the floor, fold sheets, or place a box into a car trunk. Keeping the weight close and the spine long makes these tasks safer and easier.

Safety notes for osteoporosis
Move slowly and stay within a range that lets your back remain neutral. If you feel sharp pain stop at once and resume later with a smaller range or with the wall closer behind you.

Exercise 4

Chair Sit to Stand, High Box

Purpose in plain words Train your legs and hips to rise and sit with a long neutral spine and a calm breath. This builds independence at home, helps on stairs, and prepares you for safe lifting.

Equipment Use a sturdy chair or a high box that lets you touch down without losing alignment. Wear stable shoes or go barefoot. Keep a table or rail nearby for a light touch if balance feels uncertain.

Starting position Sit near the front edge of the chair with both feet planted about hip width. Point the knees straight ahead and keep them from falling inward. Lengthen your torso so the rib cage rests above the pelvis and allow the shoulders to relax. Shift your weight slightly forward so your nose stays over your laces. Let your arms rest at your sides or crossed at the chest if you feel steady.

How to do it in calm steps Breathe in through your nose and allow the ribs to widen without lifting the chest. As you breathe out, lean the torso forward while keeping the back long. Press your feet into the floor and stand up smoothly as if you were creating gentle space between you and the seat. Once upright grow tall through the crown of the head and avoid arching the low back. Take another quiet breath. To sit down again send the pelvis back as in a small hip hinge, bend the knees, and touch the seat with control rather than dropping. Keep the spine long throughout. Repeat at the same relaxed rhythm, pairing the effort with the exhale.

Dose for beginners Complete eight controlled repetitions. Rest for about one minute and perform a second set. If this feels tiring begin with five repetitions and add one each week until you reach ten.

Progress over the weeks When the pattern is stable lower the seat by a small amount using a thinner cushion or a slightly lower chair. Build to three sets if energy allows. Later hold a light backpack close to the chest while you rise, keeping the spine long and the breath smooth. If you need an easier version place your hands lightly on your thighs to assist the first part of the stand and use a higher seat again until control returns.

Common mistakes and how to correct them Avoid throwing the torso forward to gain momentum.

Avoid rounding the back during the descent. Avoid letting the knees collapse inward. Avoid pushing the chin ahead of the body or holding your breath. If any of these appear, slow down, restart the small hip hinge, and think of pressing the floor away with your feet as you breathe out.

Carryover to daily life This same pattern supports standing from a sofa, a toilet, or a bench. It helps when you rise while holding a child or a shopping bag. Use it when you come up from gardening or after tying a shoe so the spine remains protected.

Safety notes for osteoporosis Keep the back long at every moment and move without jerks. If you feel sharp spinal pain stop, reduce the range of motion, or increase the seat height. If balance is uncertain, keep one hand near a support during the first sessions.

Exercise 5

Hip Hinge Pick Up from 30 cm Platform

Purpose in plain words
Learn to lift a light object from a raised surface while keeping the spine long and the load close. The pattern is a hip hinge with soft knees. This is the base move for picking up a bag, a small box, or a water pack without stressing the vertebrae.

Equipment
Use a firm platform about thirty centimeters high, such as a sturdy step or a stack of thick books tied together. Place a light object on the platform, for example a small backpack packed with towels or a short dumbbell. Wear stable shoes or go barefoot.

Starting position
Stand facing the object with your feet about hip width and the toes slightly open if that feels natural. Lengthen through the crown of the head, keep the shoulders wide and relaxed, and set your gaze at the horizon. Let the rib cage rest over the pelvis so the back feels long and neutral.

How to do it in calm steps

Take a gentle inhalation. Begin the hinge by sending the pelvis back. Allow the torso to tip forward just enough while the spine stays long. Bend the knees only as much as needed to reach the object. Take hold of the object and draw it immediately close to your body. Breathe out and press your feet into the floor to return to standing in one smooth motion. Think of pushing the floor away as your head grows tall. At the top remain upright without arching the low back. To put the object down repeat the same hinge in reverse and place it back on the platform with control, keeping it close to your body.

Dose for beginners

Perform six to eight smooth lifts with attention to form. Rest for a minute and complete a second set. Begin with a very light load. When the movement feels easy increase gradually to ten repetitions while keeping the breath calm.

Progress over the weeks

Increase the weight a little or reduce the platform height to twenty centimeters. Later you can lift from the floor using the same pattern. If you prefer an intermediate step, hold a small backpack close to the chest. Add progress only when the day after practice your back feels normal.

Common mistakes and how to correct them
Avoid letting the object drift away from the body. Avoid rounding the upper back. Avoid pushing the knees too far forward. Avoid holding the breath or hiking the shoulders. To correct, think pelvis back, neck long, and slide the object along the body as if it were a zipper that moves up and down close to the torso.

Carryover to daily life
Use this pattern when you collect a bag from the floor, lift a fruit crate, handle luggage, or place a box into a car trunk. Keep the weight close, hinge calmly, and breathe out during the effort.

Safety notes for osteoporosis
Avoid quick motions and twisting while holding the load. If you feel sharp back pain stop and resume later with a smaller range or lighter weight. If balance is uncertain position the platform near a stable surface so you can touch it lightly.

Exercise 6

Supported Single-Leg Stand at Counter

Purpose in plain words
Practice balance in a safe way near a stable surface. This improves control at the hips and ankles and reduces the chance of stumbles during daily life without stressing the spine.

Equipment
Use a firm counter, a sturdy table, or the back of a heavy chair. Wear shoes with a grippy sole.

Starting position
Stand facing the support with your feet about hip width. Rest the fingertips of your preferred hand lightly on the surface without leaning. Keep a long neutral spine with the rib cage resting quietly over the pelvis. Let the shoulders relax and keep your gaze level with the horizon.

How to do it in calm steps
Take an easy breath through the nose and feel the ribs widen gently to the sides. As you breathe out, shift a small portion of your weight onto the stance

leg while the torso stays upright. Lift the opposite foot a few centimeters from the floor and keep the pelvis level. Hold the position for two or three slow breaths. Feel the stance foot press the floor softly under the heel, the base of the big toe, and the base of the little toe. To finish the repetition place the lifted foot down with control and share the weight between both legs again. Repeat on the other side with the same calm rhythm.

Dose for beginners
Practice three repetitions per side and hold each for ten to fifteen seconds. Rest briefly between repetitions. Perform the drill three or four times per week at the start of a session or during quiet moments in the day.

Progress over the weeks
Reduce the pressure of the fingertips until you are only brushing the surface. Increase the hold to twenty seconds. When the stance feels steady, turn your head slowly a small amount right and left while keeping the eyes level with the horizon. Return to the simpler version whenever you feel tired.

Common mistakes and how to correct them
Avoid leaning the torso to the side to lift the foot. Avoid pulling the shoulders toward the ears. Avoid

holding your breath or bracing hard. If any of these appear, reset your stance, soften the jaw, and imagine the crown of your head growing tall while the stance foot feels the floor.

Carryover to daily life
Better balance makes you safer on uneven sidewalks, during turns in the kitchen, when stepping in and out of a tub, and when standing to put on trousers or shoes.

Safety notes for osteoporosis
Always keep a support within reach. Move slowly and with control. If you feel unsteady, place the foot down immediately and resume with a shorter hold.

Exercise 7

Heel-to-Toe Tandem Stand and Walk

Purpose in plain words
Practice a narrow base of support to improve balance and control without stressing the spine. This drill teaches the body to stay steady on curbs, narrow paths, and in crowded spaces where small adjustments matter.

Equipment
Use a clear hallway or the length of a counter so a light touch is always available. Wear shoes with a grippy sole.

Starting position
Stand tall with a long neutral spine and keep the rib cage resting over the pelvis. Place one foot directly in front of the other so the heel of the front foot touches the toes of the back foot. Let the shoulders relax and keep your gaze level with the horizon. Rest one fingertip on the counter if you need light support.

How to do it in calm steps
Take a quiet breath in through the nose and allow the ribs to widen gently to the sides. As you breathe out,

press the floor softly with both feet and notice a small natural sway while you avoid gripping your toes. Hold this tandem stance for two or three slow breaths while the back of the neck stays long. To begin walking, step the back foot forward so its heel meets the toes of the other foot. Continue with slow, small steps in a straight line. Keep the head tall and the rib cage quiet. If balance wavers, pause, place both feet side by side, breathe out, and then resume. When you reach the end of the lane, turn around with several small steps rather than a pivot and repeat in the opposite direction.

Dose for beginners
Walk eight to ten controlled steps, pause, and then complete a second pass. Practice this drill three or four times per week at the start of a session or during a calm moment of the day. If you feel unsure, begin with static holds of ten to fifteen seconds before adding steps.

Progress over the weeks
Reduce fingertip pressure until you no longer need the counter. Shorten the visual focus to a point a few meters ahead rather than looking down at the feet. Later add gentle head turns by a few degrees while

you walk, always keeping the breath smooth. Return to the simpler version on days when you feel tired.

Common mistakes and how to correct them
Avoid looking at the floor, holding the breath, lifting the shoulders, or letting the torso lean far to the side. If any of these appear, stop, stand with feet hip width, exhale slowly, and reset the tall line from crown of head to heels before trying again.

Carryover to daily life
This practice makes stepping off curbs, moving through bus or train aisles, walking in dim rooms, and turning in tight kitchens feel steadier and safer.

Safety notes for osteoporosis
Keep a support within reach and move slowly. Do not attempt quick pivots. If you feel unsteady, widen your stance immediately, breathe normally, and resume only when you feel calm and balanced.

Exercise 8

Head Turns in Single-Leg Stand

Purpose in plain words
This practice challenges your balance system gently by adding small head movements while you stand on one leg. It trains your inner ear, your eyes, and the joint sensors in your feet and hips to work together without asking your spine to bend or twist under load.

Equipment
Use a sturdy counter, a heavy chair back, or a rail that you can touch lightly. Wear shoes with a grippy sole or go barefoot on a firm surface.

Starting position
Stand tall beside the support with the rib cage resting quietly over the pelvis. Place the fingertips of one hand on the surface without leaning. Shift a little weight onto the stance leg while keeping the pelvis level and lift the other foot a few centimeters from the floor. Keep the gaze level with the horizon and lengthen the back of the neck.

How to do it in calm steps
Take an easy breath in through the nose and feel the ribs widen to the sides. As you breathe out, hold the steady single-leg stance and turn your head a small amount to the right. Pause for one calm breath without letting the shoulders creep upward or the pelvis tilt. Turn your head back to center and take another smooth breath. Now turn a small amount to the left and pause again. Keep the eyes looking straight ahead rather than down at the floor. Continue alternating gentle right and left turns for the planned time, always keeping the torso tall and quiet. If balance wavers, place the lifted foot down, reset, and begin again with a shorter hold.

Dose for beginners
Practice three rounds per side. Each round lasts ten to fifteen seconds of small head turns within a comfortable range. Rest briefly between rounds and switch stance legs. Repeat this drill three or four days per week, ideally after your warm-up breathing or posture practice.

Progress over the weeks
When the stance feels steady reduce fingertip contact until you are only brushing the surface. Increase each round to twenty seconds. Later add small up and

down nods instead of turns, always within a pain-free and comfortable range. On days when you feel tired or unsteady, return to shorter rounds with more support.

Common mistakes and how to correct them
Avoid gripping the toes or clenching the jaw. Avoid letting the shoulders rise toward the ears or letting the pelvis tip to one side. Avoid holding your breath. If any of these appear, place the foot down, exhale slowly, reset your tall line from crown of head to heel, and restart with a smaller head movement.

Carryover to daily life
Better tolerance for head turns makes crossing a street, scanning shelves in a store, and checking for traffic while stepping off a curb feel steadier. It also helps during travel when you look for signs while walking.

Safety notes for osteoporosis
Keep the spine long and the movements small. Always practice near a stable support. If you feel dizzy, stop immediately, place both feet down, breathe normally, and resume only when you feel fully steady.

Exercise 9

Step Touch Over Low Line

Purpose in plain words
This drill improves foot placement, reaction, and balance without impact. You practice clearing a small obstacle while the spine stays long and the rib cage rests quietly over the pelvis. It prepares you for uneven curbs, floor thresholds, and cluttered spaces at home and outside.

Equipment
Use a strip of tape on the floor, a thin yoga strap, or a rolled towel that creates a very low line. Stand near a counter or sturdy chair for a light touch if needed. Wear shoes with a grippy sole or go barefoot on a firm surface.

Starting position
Stand tall with your feet about hip width and the line on the floor in front of your toes. Keep your gaze level with the horizon. Let your shoulders relax. Place one hand near the support without leaning on it. Maintain a long neutral spine with the ribs resting over the pelvis.

How to do it in calm steps

Breathe in softly through the nose and allow the ribs to widen to the sides. As you breathe out, step the right foot over the line and tap the floor gently about a foot beyond it. Keep the pelvis level and the torso quiet. Step the same foot back to the starting place and feel the floor under the heel, the base of the big toe, and the base of the little toe. Repeat the same action with the left foot so the pattern becomes right then left at a smooth walking rhythm. Continue stepping and tapping over the line for the planned time. Keep the steps small and controlled rather than quick. If balance wavers, pause, place both feet side by side, exhale slowly, and resume with a lighter touch on the support.

Dose for beginners

Practice thirty to forty five seconds at a steady pace, then rest for about the same time. Complete two or three rounds. Perform this drill three or four days per week, ideally after your posture or breathing warm up.

Progress over the weeks

Move the line a little farther from your toes so the step is slightly longer. Later add a gentle change of direction by stepping over the line diagonally forward and returning to center. When this feels easy, add a light head turn to the right for a few steps and back to center, then to the left, always keeping the spine long and the breath smooth. On days when you feel tired, return to the shorter forward step with the support closer to your hand.

Common mistakes and how to correct them
Avoid looking down at the feet for the entire set. Avoid lifting the shoulders or holding the breath. Avoid turning the torso as you step. If these appear, stand tall, let the jaw soften, place your eyes on a point ahead, and imagine your head growing upward while the feet move calmly.

Carryover to daily life
The skill of clearing a low obstacle with control makes door thresholds, sidewalk cracks, and rug edges less risky. It also helps during travel when you step over suitcase straps or train gaps without rushing.

Safety notes for osteoporosis
Keep steps small and controlled. Do not attempt quick hops or large reaches. Always keep a support within reach. If you feel unsteady, widen your stance immediately, breathe normally, and resume only when you feel calm.

Exercise 10

Low Step Up with Rail

Purpose in plain words

Build leg and hip strength for stairs and curbs while keeping the spine long and quiet. This exercise improves balance and confidence during everyday transitions without impact.

Equipment

Use a low and stable step that reaches about the height of your mid shin. Keep a sturdy rail, counter, or the back of a heavy chair within easy reach. Wear shoes with a grippy sole.

Starting position

Stand facing the step with your feet about hip width. Place one hand lightly on the rail or counter if needed. Keep a long neutral spine with the rib cage resting quietly over the pelvis. Relax the shoulders and look toward the horizon so the back of the neck stays long.

How to do it in calm steps

Breathe in softly through the nose and feel the ribs widen to the sides. As you breathe out, place the whole foot of the lead leg on the step and press the step with the heel and the base of the big toe. Lean the torso a small amount forward while keeping the back long. Push through the lead foot and rise until the knee and hip extend without locking. Bring the trailing foot up to meet the lead foot on the step and stand tall for a quiet breath. To return, send the pelvis slightly back, keep the spine long, and lower the trailing foot to the floor with control. Bring the lead foot down to the floor and reset your stance before the next repetition. Keep movements smooth and match the effort to the exhale.

Dose for beginners
Perform six to eight controlled step ups on one side. Rest for about one minute and repeat on the other side. Complete two sets. If this feels heavy begin with four or five repetitions and add one repetition each week until you reach ten.

Progress over the weeks
When the pattern feels steady, reduce hand support to a light fingertip touch. Increase to three sets if energy allows. Later choose a slightly higher step or hold a small backpack close to the chest while you keep the same long spine and calm breath. On days when you feel tired or unsteady, use more support and a lower step to keep quality high.

Common mistakes and how to correct them
Avoid pushing off the back foot with a jump. Avoid letting the knee of the lead leg collapse toward the midline. Avoid rounding the back or lifting the chin toward the ceiling. If any of these appear, slow down, shift a little more weight over the lead foot before you press, and think of growing tall through the crown of the head as you stand.

Carryover to daily life
This pattern makes stairs, bus steps, and curbs feel easier. It helps when you step into a bathtub or onto a low porch and when you climb onto a small stool to reach a shelf. The same control protects the spine when you carry a light bag up a few steps.

Safety notes for osteoporosis
Move without jerks and keep the spine long at every moment. Always keep a support within reach. If you feel knee pain or sharp back pain, stop, lower the step height, or shorten the range and resume only when the movement feels comfortable and steady.

Exercise 11

Mini Band Hip Hinge with Abduction

Purpose in plain words
Teach your hips to hinge while the knees resist collapsing inward. The small outward pressure against the band builds the side hip muscles that protect the knees and pelvis. The long neutral spine keeps the vertebrae under friendly forces while you learn to bend and stand with control.

Equipment
Use a light mini band placed around both legs just above the knees. Wear stable shoes or go barefoot on a firm surface. Keep a chair back or counter within reach if balance feels uncertain.

Starting position
Stand with your feet about hip width and the toes slightly open if that feels natural. Place the mini band above your knees and create a gentle outward tension so the band is not slack. Lengthen through the crown of the head, let the shoulders rest wide, and keep the rib cage quietly stacked over the pelvis. Keep your gaze level with the horizon and the neck long.

How to do it in calm steps
Breathe in softly and feel your ribs widen to the sides. As you breathe out, send the pelvis back into a small hinge while the torso tips forward and the spine stays long. Keep the knees slightly bent and press them gently outward into the band so they remain aligned over the middle of the feet. Pause when you feel a stretch in the back of the hips and the band is under steady tension. Breathe in without lifting the chest. As you breathe out again, press the feet into the floor and return to standing in one smooth motion. Finish tall without arching the low back. Maintain the same light outward pressure on the band through the entire movement. Move slowly so the band does not snap the knees inward.

Dose for beginners
Perform eight controlled repetitions. Rest for about one minute and complete a second set. If this feels easy, build to ten repetitions while keeping the same calm breath and careful alignment.

Progress over the weeks
When the pattern feels steady choose a slightly firmer band or hold a small backpack close to the chest so the hips work a bit more. Later hinge a little deeper while the spine remains long and the band

tension stays steady. On days when you feel tired or your knees drift inward, return to the lighter band and a smaller range until control returns.

Common mistakes and how to correct them
Avoid letting the band pull the knees together. Avoid rounding the upper back or pushing the chin forward. Avoid shifting the weight to the toes. If these appear, think of sitting the pelvis back, keeping the neck long, and pressing the knees outward just enough to align over the middle of the feet. Keep the weight shared between heel and forefoot.

Carryover to daily life
Stronger side hips and a clear hinge make standing from low seats, lifting a grocery bag, loading a washer, or getting a suitcase off the floor feel steadier. The knees stay in line and the spine remains long while the work shifts to the hips where it is safer.

Safety notes for osteoporosis
Move slowly and keep a neutral spine at all times. Do not force deep ranges. If you feel sharp pain in the back or knees, stop and resume later with a lighter band and a shorter hinge. Keep a support within reach if balance is uncertain.

Exercise 12

Bridge on Floor, Neutral Spine

Purpose in plain words
Strengthen the back of the hips and thighs while the spine stays long and quiet. This teaches the body to share load through the hips instead of the lower back and prepares you for safer lifts and stairs.

Equipment
Use a firm mat or carpet. Wear shoes with a grippy sole or go barefoot.

Starting position
Lie on your back with the knees bent and the feet about hip width. Place the feet so you can just touch your heels with your fingertips. Rest the arms by your sides with the palms down. Let the rib cage settle toward the pelvis so the lower back feels natural rather than pressed flat. Lengthen the back of the neck and look straight up so the throat stays soft.

How to do it in calm steps
Breathe in through the nose and feel the ribs widen gently to the sides. As you breathe out, press the feet into the floor and imagine drawing the floor toward

you with the heels. Let the pelvis float upward a little at a time until the hips open to a straight line from shoulders to knees. Keep the ribs quiet and avoid pushing them toward the ceiling. Hold the top for one soft breath while the glutes stay firm and the neck remains long. Lower the pelvis slowly, keeping the spine quiet, and return the sacrum to the mat with control. Pause for a moment, breathe in, and begin the next repetition with the same smooth rhythm. If the hamstrings cramp, move the feet a little farther from the hips and think of gently squeezing the glutes before you lift.

Dose for beginners
Perform eight calm repetitions. Rest for about one minute and complete a second set. If this feels heavy start with five repetitions and add one repetition each week until you reach ten.

Progress over the weeks
When the pattern feels steady pause for two slow breaths at the top of each lift. Later place a light miniband around the thighs just above the knees and keep a gentle outward pressure as you bridge so the knees stay aligned. You can also elevate the feet on a low step to change the angle once you are comfortable. On days when you feel tired or the

lower back feels sensitive, reduce the range and hold a shorter top position until comfort returns.

Common mistakes and how to correct them
Avoid arching the lower back at the top. Avoid flaring the ribs or pushing the chin upward. Avoid letting the knees drift together. If these appear, lower a little, exhale softly, think of length from knees to shoulders, and keep a light outward tension at the thighs so the knees remain over the middle of the feet.

Carryover to daily life
Stronger hips make standing from a chair, climbing stairs, walking up slopes, and lifting a light bag from the floor feel steadier. The spine remains protected while the hips do more of the work.

Safety notes for osteoporosis
Move smoothly without jerks. Keep a neutral spine through the lift and avoid end range arching. If you feel sharp back pain or dizziness, stop, rest, and resume only with a smaller range or after speaking with your clinician.

Exercise 13

Supported Split Squat Short Stance

Purpose in plain words
Build strength in the thighs and hips while you keep a long neutral spine. The short stance reduces pressure and allows you to control balance. This pattern prepares you for stairs, rising from lower seats, and lifting tasks where one leg works more than the other.

Equipment
Use a sturdy counter, rail, or the back of a heavy chair for a light touch. Wear shoes with a grippy sole.

Starting position
Stand tall with your feet hip width. Step one foot forward about the length of a small stride and keep the back heel lifted. Place two fingertips on the support with the hand that feels natural. Keep your rib cage resting over the pelvis and let the shoulders relax. Look toward the horizon so the back of the neck stays long.

How to do it in calm steps
Breathe in softly through the nose and let the ribs

widen toward the sides. As you breathe out, send the pelvis slightly back and allow both knees to bend a small amount. Lower your body until the front thigh feels work but the back knee stays a comfortable distance from the floor. Keep the torso tall and quiet. The front knee stays aligned over the middle of the foot and does not collapse inward. Pause at the bottom for a soft breath without lifting the chest. Breathe out again and press the front foot into the floor to rise in one smooth motion. Finish tall without arching the low back. Reset your stance and repeat the same calm rhythm for the planned number of repetitions before changing sides.

Dose for beginners
Perform six to eight controlled repetitions on the first side. Rest about one minute. Perform the same number on the second side. Complete two sets. If this feels heavy begin with four or five repetitions and add one each week until you reach ten.

Progress over the weeks
Reduce hand support to a light fingertip touch. Increase to three sets if energy allows. Later hold a small backpack close to the chest to add a little load while keeping the same long spine and quiet ribs. You can also increase the range slightly by lowering

a little deeper as comfort allows. On days when balance feels unsure, shorten the stride and use more support to keep quality high.

Common mistakes and how to correct them
Avoid tipping the torso forward or rounding the back. Avoid pushing the front knee inward or letting it slide far beyond the toes. Avoid holding your breath. If any of these appear, slow down, keep the eyes level, think of the crown of the head growing upward, and press the front foot evenly through heel and forefoot during the rise.

Carryover to daily life
This exercise makes getting up from lower chairs, stepping onto a curb, climbing stairs, and carrying a small bag or child feel more organised and stable. The hips share the work and the spine remains protected.

Safety notes for osteoporosis
Move slowly and avoid jerks. Keep a neutral spine at every moment. If you feel sharp pain in the back or knees, stop, reduce the range or shorten the stance, and resume only when the movement feels comfortable and steady.

Exercise 14

Side-Lying Hip Abduction

Purpose in plain words
Strengthen the side hip muscles that keep the pelvis stable during walking and stairs. This support reduces wobble and protects the spine by improving control at the hips.

Equipment
Use a firm mat or carpet. A small folded towel can support the head. Wear comfortable clothing that allows the leg to move freely.

Starting position
Lie on your side with the bottom arm bent so your head rests on the forearm or on a small towel. Keep the body in a straight line from head to heels. Bend the bottom knee slightly for stability. Straighten the top leg in line with the torso and point the toes forward so the kneecap faces ahead. Place the top hand on the floor in front of your chest for light balance. Keep the rib cage resting quietly over the pelvis and the neck long.

How to do it in calm steps
Take a quiet breath in through the nose and let the ribs widen gently. As you breathe out, lift the straight top leg slowly a small distance toward the ceiling while the pelvis stays still and the toes point forward. Stop when you feel the side of the hip working without rolling the body backward. Hold the top position for one soft breath while the neck remains long. Lower the leg with control until it almost touches the other leg, then begin the next repetition with the same smooth rhythm. Keep the movement small and slow so the side hip muscles do the work rather than momentum.

Dose for beginners
Perform eight calm repetitions on the first side. Rest briefly, turn to the other side, and repeat the same number. Complete two sets. If this feels heavy begin with five repetitions and add one each week until you reach ten.

Progress over the weeks
When the pattern feels steady pause for two slow breaths at the top of each lift. Later place a light miniband around both ankles and keep the same alignment while lifting. You can also draw small controlled circles at the top position for a few

seconds to increase time under tension. On days when the hip feels tired or the low back feels sensitive, return to the basic version without band and with a smaller range.

Common mistakes and how to correct them
Avoid rolling the pelvis backward or turning the toes toward the ceiling. Avoid hiking the top hip toward the ribs or gripping the neck and shoulders. If these appear, lower a little, point the toes forward again, lengthen through the crown of the head, and think of reaching the heel away from you as you lift.

Carryover to daily life
Stronger side hips make walking feel smoother, help you stay steady on uneven ground, and reduce knee collapse when you rise from chairs or climb stairs. The spine stays quieter because the pelvis does not tip side to side.

Safety notes for osteoporosis
Move slowly without jerks and keep the torso in a straight line. Do not hold your breath. If you feel sharp pain in the back or in the front of the hip, stop and resume later with a shorter range or after checking your setup.

Exercise 15

Seated Marches with Neutral Spine

Purpose in plain words
Wake up the hip flexors and deep trunk support without rounding the back. This drill builds control for walking, stair starts, and getting into cars while keeping the spine calm.

Equipment
Use a sturdy chair without wheels. Wear stable shoes or go barefoot so you feel the floor.

Starting position
Sit near the front edge of the chair. Place both feet flat and about hip width apart. Rest your hands lightly on the sides of the seat or on your thighs. Grow tall through the crown of the head so the rib cage rests quietly over the pelvis. Keep the shoulders relaxed and the gaze level with the horizon. The lower back should feel natural rather than pressed flat.

How to do it in calm steps
Breathe in through the nose and allow the ribs to widen gently toward the sides. As you breathe out,

press the right foot softly into the floor and lift the left foot a few centimeters as if beginning a small march. Keep the torso tall and quiet. Hold the lifted foot for a slow count of one, place it down with control, and breathe in again. Breathe out and switch sides by pressing the left foot into the floor and lifting the right foot a few centimeters. Continue alternating side to side at a steady rhythm. Keep the movement small and smooth so the pelvis stays level and the spine remains long. If the shoulders creep toward the ears, pause, relax them downward, and resume with a slower pace.

Dose for beginners
March for thirty to forty five seconds, then rest for about the same time. Complete two or three rounds. Practice this drill three or four days per week, ideally after your breathing or posture warm up.

Progress over the weeks
Hold each lifted foot for a longer pause before setting it down. Place a light miniband around the ankles for gentle resistance while you keep the same tall posture. Later lift each knee a little higher without letting the back round. On days when you feel tired or your back feels sensitive, keep the lift very small and the holds short so quality stays high.

Common mistakes and how to correct them
Avoid leaning backward or slumping forward. Avoid rocking side to side on the chair. Avoid lifting the chin or holding your breath. If these appear, reset the tall line from crown of head to pelvis, keep the gaze level, and think of growing upward as the leg moves.

Carryover to daily life
This practice makes the first step away from a chair, the start of a stair climb, and getting into a car feel more organised. Hips and trunk share the work while the spine stays protected.

Safety notes for osteoporosis
Move slowly and keep a neutral spine throughout. Do not force large lifts. If you feel sharp back pain or dizziness, stop and resume later with a smaller range or after speaking with your clinician.

Exercise 16

Band Row at Chest Height

Purpose in plain words
Strengthen the muscles of the upper back and teach the shoulders to glide while the rib cage stays quiet and the spine remains long. This pattern supports posture, improves pulling strength for daily tasks, and protects the neck and lower back.

Equipment
Use a long resistance band anchored at chest height to a solid point such as a closed door with a safe anchor, a heavy railing, or a sturdy post. Wear stable shoes and stand on a firm surface.

Starting position
Stand facing the anchor with the feet about hip width and the knees softly unlocked. Hold one end of the band in each hand with the palms facing each other. Step back until there is light tension in the band with the arms extended in front of you. Stack the ribs over the pelvis and let the shoulders rest wide. Keep the gaze level with the horizon and lengthen the back of the neck so the crown of the head grows tall.

How to do it in calm steps
Breathe in through the nose and allow the ribs to widen gently to the sides without lifting the chest. As you breathe out, press the feet into the floor and draw the elbows back toward your sides while the forearms remain parallel to the floor. Think of the shoulder blades gliding toward the spine rather than the shoulders hiking toward the ears. Pause for one soft breath with the band close to your ribs and the torso quiet. Breathe out again as you return the arms forward with control until the elbows are straight but not locked. Keep the neck long and the ribs settled so the low back does not arch. Continue with the same smooth rhythm, matching each pull to the exhale and each return to an easy inhale.

Dose for beginners
Perform eight controlled repetitions. Rest for about one minute and complete a second set. If this feels easy build to ten repetitions while keeping the same calm breath and steady posture.

Progress over the weeks
Step a little farther from the anchor to increase tension or choose a slightly firmer band. Later perform the row in a small split stance so the front to back balance improves while the spine stays long.

You can also pause for two slow breaths at the end of the pull to build endurance between the shoulder blades. On days when the neck or low back feels sensitive, move closer to the anchor and reduce tension so form stays crisp.

Common mistakes and how to correct them
Avoid shrugging the shoulders toward the ears, arching the low back, flaring the ribs, or snapping the band forward. If any of these appear, soften the knees, exhale gently, think of the shoulder blades sliding down and back, and keep the crown of the head reaching upward. The hands travel toward the lower ribs rather than the throat so the neck remains free.

Carryover to daily life
A steady row pattern helps with pulling a heavy door, stabilizing a backpack on the shoulders, lifting a suitcase handle, and maintaining an open chest posture during long walks or travel. The upper back does more work and the neck and low back are spared.

Safety notes for osteoporosis
Keep the spine neutral and the movement slow. Do not lean far back to create resistance. Inspect the anchor before each session and replace worn bands.

If you feel sharp pain in the shoulder or back, stop, reset the posture, and resume only with lighter tension.

Exercise 17

Seated Band Lat Pull to Collarbone

Purpose in plain words
Build strength in the large back muscles while keeping the neck relaxed and the rib cage quiet. This pull supports posture, helps with overhead reach in daily life, and protects the lower back by teaching the torso to stay long and steady.

Equipment
Use a long resistance band anchored above head height to a solid point such as the top of a closed door with a safe anchor or a sturdy beam. Sit on a stable chair without wheels. Wear shoes with a grippy sole.

Starting position
Sit near the front edge of the chair with both feet planted about hip width. Hold one end of the band in each hand with the palms facing forward. Reach the arms comfortably toward the anchor so there is light tension in the band. Stack the ribs over the pelvis so the back feels long and neutral. Let the shoulders rest wide and keep the gaze level with the horizon.

Lengthen the back of the neck so the crown of the head grows tall.

How to do it in calm steps
Breathe in through the nose and allow the ribs to widen gently to the sides without lifting the chest. As you breathe out, press the feet into the floor and pull the elbows down and slightly backward toward the sides of the rib cage. Guide the hands toward the line of the collarbones rather than toward the throat. Think of the shoulder blades sliding down and in toward the spine while the neck stays long and relaxed. Pause for one soft breath in the bottom position. Breathe out again and return the arms upward with control until the elbows are straight but not locked and the band has light tension. Keep the torso quiet and avoid arching the lower back. Continue with the same smooth rhythm, pairing each pull with the exhale and each return with an easy inhale.

Dose for beginners
Perform eight calm repetitions. Rest for about one minute and complete a second set. If this feels easy, build to ten repetitions while keeping the same steady posture and breath.

Progress over the weeks
Move the chair a little farther from the anchor to increase tension or choose a slightly firmer band. Later hold the bottom position for two slow breaths to build endurance between the shoulder blades. You can also try a small staggered stance with one foot slightly ahead to challenge trunk control while the spine remains long. On days when the neck or back feels sensitive, sit closer to the anchor and reduce tension so form stays crisp.

Common mistakes and how to correct them
Avoid shrugging the shoulders toward the ears. Avoid pulling the bar path toward the face. Avoid flaring the ribs or arching the lower back. If any of these appear, soften the knees and exhale gently, think of the shoulder blades sliding down your back, and let the hands travel toward the collarbone line while the crown of the head reaches upward.

Carryover to daily life
A strong and well timed lat pull helps with lowering objects from a shelf, closing a heavy hatch, steadying a backpack on the shoulders, and keeping an open chest posture during longer walks or travel.

Safety notes for osteoporosis
Keep the spine neutral and move slowly. Do not lean

far back to create resistance. Inspect the anchor before each session and replace worn bands. If you feel sharp pain in the shoulders or back, stop, reset your posture, and resume only with lighter tension or after speaking with your clinician.

Exercise 18

Wall Push Up

Purpose in plain words
Build pushing strength for chest, shoulders, and arms while keeping the spine long and the rib cage quiet. This version reduces load compared with floor push ups and lets you learn control without stress on the lower back or wrists.

Equipment
Use a clear wall that does not slip. Wear shoes with a grippy sole.

Starting position
Stand facing the wall at about one full step away. Place your hands on the wall at chest height and a little wider than shoulder width. Spread the fingers and let the palms settle flat. Walk the feet back or forward until your body forms a straight line from head to heels. Keep the knees softly unlocked, the rib cage resting over the pelvis, and the back of the neck long. Look slightly downward so the head follows the line of the spine.

How to do it in calm steps
Breathe in through the nose and allow the ribs to widen gently without lifting the chest. As you breathe out, press the hands into the wall and feel the shoulders slide down your back. Inhale again and bend the elbows so the body moves toward the wall in one piece. Keep the torso long and quiet and let the elbows travel about forty five degrees from the ribs rather than flaring straight out. Stop when your chest is a few centimeters from the wall and the shoulder blades feel connected. Breathe out and press the wall away, straightening the elbows without locking and returning to the tall line. Continue at a steady rhythm, matching the press to the exhale and the lower to a quiet inhale.

Dose for beginners
Perform eight calm repetitions. Rest for about one minute and complete a second set. If this feels easy build to ten repetitions while keeping the same smooth form.

Progress over the weeks
Step the feet a little farther from the wall to increase the angle and the load while keeping the body in a straight line. Later place your hands on the back of a sturdy chair or countertop to move to an incline

version. You can also pause for two slow breaths near the wall before pressing back to build control. On days when the neck or wrists feel sensitive, reduce the angle by stepping closer and keep the range smaller.

Common mistakes and how to correct them
Avoid letting the lower back arch or the ribs flare forward. Avoid shrugging the shoulders toward the ears. Avoid dropping the head or letting the elbows flare straight out to the sides. If any of these appear, reset the tall line from crown of head to heels, soften the knees, and think of the shoulder blades gliding down and in as you press.

Carryover to daily life
Stronger pushing helps with closing heavy doors, transferring from the floor to hands and knees, rising from a countertop lean, and controlling a shopping cart without straining the back.

Safety notes for osteoporosis
Keep movements slow and the spine neutral. Do not bounce at the wall or hold your breath. If you feel sharp pain in the shoulders, wrists, or back, stop and resume later with a smaller range, a closer stance, or advice from your clinician.

Exercise 19

Seated Dumbbell Press to Eye Level

Purpose in plain words
Build shoulder and upper back strength while keeping the rib cage quiet and the spine long. Stopping the press at eye level protects the neck and the lower back and avoids end range strain. This pattern supports safer reaching in daily life.

Equipment
Use a sturdy chair without wheels and a pair of light dumbbells or two equal household objects such as small water bottles. Wear shoes with a grippy sole.

Starting position
Sit near the front edge of the chair with both feet planted about hip width. Hold a weight in each hand and bring them to shoulder height with the palms facing forward or slightly inward. Stack the ribs softly over the pelvis so the lower back feels natural rather than arched. Let the shoulders rest wide and keep your gaze level with the horizon. Lengthen the back of the neck so the crown of the head grows tall.

How to do it in calm steps
Breathe in through the nose and allow the ribs to widen gently toward the sides. As you breathe out, press the weights upward along a slight forward path until your hands reach the line of your eyes. Keep the elbows slightly in front of the body rather than flaring straight out. Pause for a soft breath at eye level while the shoulders stay down and the neck remains long. Breathe out again and lower the weights with control to the starting position at the shoulders. Keep the rib cage settled and avoid leaning back or lifting the chest. Continue at a steady rhythm and match each press to the exhale and each return to a quiet inhale.

Dose for beginners
Perform eight controlled repetitions. Rest for about one minute and complete a second set. If this feels easy build to ten repetitions while keeping the same smooth form. Choose a load that feels light to moderate so the last two repetitions are effortful but steady.

Progress over the weeks
Increase the weight in small steps when both sets feel comfortable and your form remains calm the next day. You can also pause for two slow breaths at eye

level to build control around the shoulder blades. Another option is to press one arm at a time while the other hand holds at shoulder height which challenges trunk control. On days when the neck or back feels sensitive choose lighter weights or perform the movement with no load and focus on the path and breath.

Common mistakes and how to correct them
Avoid arching the lower back or letting the ribs flare forward. Avoid shrugging the shoulders toward the ears or pushing the chin upward. Avoid lowering the weights quickly. If any of these appear reset your tall posture press more forward than straight up keep the neck long and move more slowly. If the weights pull you backward sit a little more upright and bring the elbows slightly in front of the body before starting the next repetition.

Carryover to daily life
Stronger and better controlled shoulders make it easier to place light items onto eye level shelves close a heavy hatch push a window open and support a child at chest height without straining the back.

Safety notes for osteoporosis
Keep the range to eye level rather than overhead. Maintain a neutral spine. Avoid holding your breath.

If you feel sharp pain in the shoulder or back stop and resume later with a lighter load or after speaking with your clinician.

Exercise 20

Band Chest Press in Split Stance

Purpose in plain words
Strengthen the chest, shoulders, and arms while the trunk stays steady and the rib cage remains quiet. The split stance teaches your body to resist being pulled backward by the band, which builds safe front-to-back control without stressing the spine.

Equipment
Use a long resistance band anchored behind you at chest height to a solid point such as a closed door with a safe anchor or a sturdy post. Wear shoes with a grippy sole and stand on a firm surface.

Starting position
Stand facing away from the anchor and hold one end of the band in each hand. Step one foot forward and one foot back into a comfortable split stance with both feet pointing ahead. Keep a slight bend in both knees. Bring the hands to chest level with the elbows gently in front of the body. Stack the ribs over the pelvis so the lower back feels natural rather than arched. Let the shoulders rest wide and keep your

gaze level with the horizon. Lengthen the back of the neck so the crown of the head grows tall.

How to do it in calm steps
Breathe in through the nose and allow the ribs to widen to the sides. As you breathe out, press both hands forward until the elbows are straight but not locked. Keep the hands traveling along a path in front of the chest rather than drifting upward. Pause for a soft breath with the arms long while the trunk stays quiet and the back heel presses gently into the floor for stability. Breathe out again and return the hands to the chest with control, letting the shoulder blades glide back without lifting the chest or arching the lower back. Continue with this smooth rhythm and feel the front leg share the work with the trunk. After the planned number of repetitions, switch the stance so the other foot is forward and repeat.

Dose for beginners
Perform eight calm presses with the left foot forward, then rest briefly and repeat eight presses with the right foot forward. Complete two sets. If this feels easy build to ten repetitions per side while keeping the same steady posture and breath.

Progress over the weeks
Step a little farther from the anchor to increase band

tension or choose a slightly firmer band. Pause for two slow breaths at the end of the press to build control. Later press one arm at a time while the other hand holds at the chest, which challenges trunk stability without changing the spine position. On days when the neck or low back feels sensitive, move closer to the anchor and reduce tension so form stays crisp.

Common mistakes and how to correct them
Avoid flaring the ribs or arching the lower back. Avoid shrugging the shoulders toward the ears. Avoid letting the hands travel high toward the face or dropping the head forward. If any of these appear, soften the knees, exhale gently, keep the hands at chest height, and imagine the shoulder blades sliding down and around the rib cage as you press.

Carryover to daily life
A steady band press helps with closing heavy doors, pushing a shopping cart, guiding a suitcase, and supporting a child at chest height without straining the back. The trunk learns to stay quiet while the arms do the work.

Safety notes for osteoporosis
Keep the spine neutral and movements slow. Do not lean far forward to create force. Inspect the anchor

before each session and replace worn bands. If you feel sharp pain in the shoulders or back, stop, reset your posture, and resume only with lighter tension.

Exercise 21

Farmer Carry with Light Dumbbells

Purpose in plain words
Practice walking tall while carrying weight close to the body. This builds grip, shoulder stability, and trunk control that protect the spine during daily tasks like carrying groceries or moving a small suitcase.

Equipment
Use two light dumbbells or two equal household objects with handles. Wear shoes with a grippy sole and choose a clear lane of six to ten meters.

Starting position
Stand tall with a long neutral spine and let the rib cage rest quietly over the pelvis. Hold one weight in each hand with the arms at your sides and the palms facing the thighs. Keep the shoulders relaxed and slightly back so the collarbones feel wide. Look toward the horizon so the back of the neck stays long. Set the feet about hip width and feel equal pressure under heel, big toe base, and little toe base.

How to do it in calm steps
Breathe in softly through the nose and allow the ribs

to widen toward the sides. As you breathe out, press the floor away and begin walking at a measured pace. Keep the weights close to the thighs rather than swinging them far forward. Let the shoulder blades sit low and glide gently as you move. Maintain a quiet torso without leaning backward or side to side. Walk the planned distance, turn around with several small steps rather than a pivot, and return to the starting point with the same tall posture. Set the weights down using a small hip hinge so the back remains long and the load stays close to your body.

Dose for beginners
Walk for two passes of six to ten meters with a short rest between passes. Complete two rounds. Choose a load that feels easy at first so posture stays calm and the breath remains smooth. When this is comfortable, extend each pass by a few meters before increasing weight.

Progress over the weeks
Increase distance gradually or add small amounts of weight while preserving the tall line and quiet ribs. Later use a gentle tempo change by walking slightly slower for a few steps to build control. When the pattern feels steady, practice a careful turn around a cone or chair using short steps while the shoulders

stay down. On days when the neck or lower back feels sensitive, reduce the load and shorten the distance so quality remains high.

Common mistakes and how to correct them
Avoid gripping the weights with stiff elbows or hiking the shoulders toward the ears. Avoid leaning backward, letting the ribs flare, or letting the head poke forward. If any of these appear, pause, set the weights down safely with a hinge, reset your posture, and continue with a lighter load or shorter distance. Think of growing tall through the crown of the head and letting the arms hang heavy and quiet at the sides.

Carryover to daily life
This pattern makes carrying shopping bags, water bottles, gardening tools, or a small suitcase feel steadier and safer. The trunk learns to resist sway and the spine stays protected while the hips and legs do the work.

Safety notes for osteoporosis
Choose light weights and move slowly. Keep the load close to the body and use a hip hinge when picking up or setting down. If you feel sharp pain in the back, shoulders, or hands, stop and resume later

with a lighter load or after speaking with your clinician.

Exercise 22

Suitcase Carry One Side

Purpose in plain words
Practice walking tall while carrying weight on one side only. This teaches the trunk to resist leaning and builds shoulder and grip strength. It prepares you for daily tasks like carrying a single shopping bag or moving a small suitcase without stressing the spine.

Equipment
Use one light dumbbell or a small bag with a secure handle. Wear shoes with a good grip. Choose a clear lane of six to ten meters.

Starting position
Stand tall and hold the weight in one hand at your side. Let the arm hang straight with a relaxed elbow. Keep the rib cage resting quietly over the pelvis so the lower back feels natural. Set your gaze at the horizon and lengthen the back of the neck. Place the feet about hip width and feel even pressure under heel, base of the big toe, and base of the little toe. Let the free arm hang quietly or brush the thigh.

How to do it in calm steps
Take a quiet breath in through the nose and feel the ribs widen gently to the sides. As you breathe out, press the floor away and begin to walk at a measured pace. Keep the weight close to your thigh and avoid letting it swing forward. Imagine a tall line from crown of head to heel and keep the shoulders level. Walk the planned distance, turn around with several small steps rather than a quick pivot, and return to the start with the same calm posture. Set the weight down using a small hip hinge so the back stays long and the load remains close. Switch hands and repeat on the other side.

Dose for beginners
Walk two passes of six to ten meters with the weight in the right hand, then rest briefly and do the same with the weight in the left hand. Complete two rounds. Choose a light load that allows a smooth breath and a steady tall posture.

Progress over the weeks
Increase distance a little at a time or add a small amount of weight while keeping the same posture. Later practice short pauses during the walk where you stand still for two calm breaths before moving again. You can also practice a gentle change of

direction around a chair using short steps while the shoulders stay level. On days when the neck or lower back feels sensitive, use a lighter load and shorten the distance so quality remains high.

Common mistakes and how to correct them
Avoid leaning away from the weight or letting the rib cage flare forward. Avoid hiking the shoulder toward the ear or gripping the handle so hard that the forearm tenses. Avoid long strides that pull the trunk side to side. If any of these appear, pause and set the weight down with a hinge, reset your tall posture, relax the shoulders, and continue with a lighter load or a shorter path.

Carryover to daily life
A steady suitcase carry makes it easier to hold a single grocery bag, guide a small suitcase, carry a watering can, or lift a modest object from a shelf and walk with it while the spine remains protected.

Safety notes for osteoporosis
Keep the load close to the body and move slowly. Use a hip hinge to pick up and set down the weight. If you feel sharp pain in the back, shoulder, or hand, stop and resume later with a lighter load or after speaking with your clinician.

Exercise 23

Front Load Carry with Backpack

Purpose in plain words
Practice walking tall while hugging a light load close to your chest. This teaches the trunk to stay steady and the hips to do the work, which protects the spine during daily lifts and short carries.

Equipment
Use an empty backpack or a small duffel. Place a few towels or light items inside so the load is modest and the shape is soft. Wear shoes with a good grip and choose a clear lane of six to ten meters.

Starting position
Stand tall and place the backpack against your chest with the bottom of the bag resting above the belt line. Wrap both forearms around the bag as if you were holding a sleeping cat. Keep the elbows slightly down and close to the ribs. Set the rib cage quietly over the pelvis so the lower back feels natural. Let the shoulders rest wide. Keep the gaze level with the horizon and lengthen the back of the neck.

How to do it in calm steps
Take a quiet breath in through the nose and let the ribs widen to the sides. As you breathe out, press the floor away and begin walking at a measured pace. Keep the bag close so it touches the body without bouncing. Allow small relaxed arm pressure rather than a hard squeeze. Maintain a quiet torso without leaning backward or looking down. Walk the planned distance, turn with several short steps rather than a quick pivot, and return to the start with the same tall posture. To put the bag down, stop, set your feet, breathe out, hinge the hips a little, and slide the bag onto a table or chair rather than the floor so the spine stays long.

Dose for beginners
Walk two passes of six to ten meters, rest for about the same time, then complete a second round. Choose a load that lets you keep a smooth breath and easy posture from start to finish. Build distance before you add weight.

Progress over the weeks
Increase distance a little or add a small amount of weight while keeping the same calm posture. Later practice a gentle stop and start by pausing for one soft breath every three or four steps and then walking

on. You can also practice a shallow step up onto a very low platform during the carry once the basic walk feels steady. On days when the neck or lower back feels sensitive, use a lighter bag and shorten the distance so quality remains high.

Common mistakes and how to correct them
Avoid arching the lower back or flaring the ribs forward. Avoid lifting the chin or pulling the shoulders toward the ears. Avoid squeezing the bag so hard that the breath becomes shallow. If these appear, stop, place the bag on a table with a small hip hinge, reset your tall posture, soften the shoulders, and continue with a lighter load or a shorter path.

Carryover to daily life
This pattern makes carrying a small parcel, holding a baby close to the chest, or moving a stack of folded towels feel steadier. The load stays near your center, the hips drive the movement, and the spine remains protected.

Safety notes for osteoporosis
Keep the load light and close. Move slowly and turn with short steps. Use a hip hinge when setting the bag down and choose a higher surface when possible. If you feel sharp pain in the back or chest, stop and

resume later with a lighter load or after speaking with your clinician.

Exercise 24

Grocery Bag Lift and Carry Drill

Purpose in plain words
Practice the full sequence of approaching, lifting, turning, and walking with a light bag while the spine stays long and the load remains close. This turns everyday shopping into a safe pattern that protects the back and hips.

Equipment
Use a reusable grocery bag or a small tote with comfortable handles. Place a few lightweight items inside such as towels, fruit, or water bottles. Wear shoes with a grippy sole and choose a clear area with a table or counter nearby.

Starting position
Stand tall with the bag on a low platform such as a small step or a box. Keep the feet about hip width and the toes slightly open if that feels natural. Let the rib cage rest quietly over the pelvis so the back feels long. Set your gaze toward the horizon and allow the shoulders to relax.

How to do it in calm steps

Begin a few short paces from the bag and walk toward it at an easy pace. Stop with the shins close to the edge of the platform. Take a quiet breath in through the nose. As you breathe out, send the pelvis back into a small hip hinge and let the torso tip forward while the spine stays long. Bend the knees only as much as needed. Slide both hands to the handles and draw the bag close to your shins before you lift. Exhale and press the feet into the floor to rise in one smooth motion, keeping the bag against the body so the arms feel light. Stand tall for one soft breath. To turn, take several short steps while facing the new direction rather than twisting the torso. Begin walking at a measured pace with the bag close to your side or held at the chest if the handles are short. After a few meters stop, exhale, hinge a little, and place the bag onto a table or counter so the spine stays long. Pause for a calm breath and repeat the sequence from a new angle.

Dose for beginners

Practice three to five full cycles of approach, lift, turn, walk, and set down. Rest for about one minute between cycles. Begin with a very light bag so posture and breath stay calm. Repeat this drill two or three times per week.

Progress over the weeks
Add a small amount of weight to the bag while preserving the same smooth rhythm. Increase the walking distance a little or include a shallow step up onto a low platform before setting the bag down on a counter. When the pattern feels natural, alternate sides by carrying the bag on the left during one cycle and on the right during the next. On days when the back feels sensitive, keep the bag very light and shorten the path so quality remains high.

Common mistakes and how to correct them
Avoid lifting the bag with straight legs and a rounded back. Avoid letting the bag swing away from the body during the rise. Avoid turning the torso while holding the bag at arm's length. If any of these appear, reset your stance, bring the bag close before you lift, hinge from the hips, and turn with several short steps while the spine remains quiet.

Carryover to daily life
This drill mirrors real tasks such as loading groceries into a car, moving a laundry basket, or carrying a parcel to the door. Keeping the load close and the spine long makes these moments feel safer and more organised.

Safety notes for osteoporosis
Move slowly and match effort to a gentle exhale. Keep the load close at all times and avoid quick twists. Choose a table or counter for setting the bag down so you do not have to reach to the floor. Stop if you feel sharp pain and resume later with a lighter bag or after speaking with your clinician.

Exercise 25

Step Down Control from Low Step

Purpose in plain words
Learn to come down from a small step with steady hips, quiet ribs, and a long spine. This builds the eccentric strength that protects knees and hips and keeps the back calm on stairs and curbs.

Equipment
Use a low and stable step about mid shin height. Keep a sturdy rail, counter, or the back of a heavy chair within easy reach. Wear shoes with a good grip.

Starting position
Stand on the step with both feet. Place one hand lightly on the rail or counter if you need a touch for balance. Keep a long neutral spine and let the rib cage rest quietly over the pelvis. Relax the shoulders and look toward the horizon so the back of the neck stays long. Choose a lead leg that will stay on the step while the other leg steps to the floor.

How to do it in calm steps
Breathe in softly through the nose and feel the ribs widen to the sides. As you breathe out, send the

pelvis slightly back and let the torso tip a little forward while the spine stays long. Slide the free foot slowly toward the floor and touch the heel down with control. Keep most of your weight over the foot that remains on the step. Pause for a soft breath with both feet in contact and the knees gently bent. Breathe out again and press through the foot on the step to return the free foot back up onto the step without a hop. Stand tall at the top for a calm breath and repeat the same rhythm. After you complete the planned number of repetitions, switch the lead leg so both sides train evenly.

Dose for beginners
Perform six to eight controlled step downs on one side. Rest for about one minute. Perform the same number on the other side. Complete two sets. If this feels heavy begin with four or five repetitions and add one each week until you reach ten.

Progress over the weeks
Reduce hand support to a light fingertip touch. Increase to three sets if energy allows. Later use a slightly higher step or hold a small backpack close to the chest while you keep the same long spine and quiet breath. On days when the knees or back feel

sensitive, return to a lower step and a smaller range so quality remains high.

Common mistakes and how to correct them
Avoid dropping quickly to the floor. Avoid letting the knee of the stance leg collapse toward the midline. Avoid rounding the back or lifting the chin. If any of these appear, slow down, keep the eyes level, press the stance foot evenly through heel and forefoot, and imagine the crown of the head growing upward as you return to the top.

Carryover to daily life
This pattern makes down stairs, bus steps, curbs, and small drops in the garden feel easier and safer. It also helps when you carry a light bag down a short flight because the hips control the descent and the spine remains protected.

Safety notes for osteoporosis
Move without jerks and keep the spine long at every moment. Always keep a support within reach. If you feel knee pain or sharp back pain, stop, lower the step height, or shorten the range and resume only when the movement feels comfortable and steady.

Exercise 26

Dead Bug Heel Taps

Purpose in plain words
Teach the trunk to stay quiet while the legs move. This builds deep support for the spine without curling the back. The pattern helps you control everyday tasks such as standing from a chair, walking with bags, and stepping off a curb.

Equipment
Use a firm mat or carpet. Wear comfortable clothing that allows the hips to move freely.

Starting position
Lie on your back and let the rib cage settle so the lower back feels natural rather than pressed flat. Bring both hips and knees to a tabletop shape with the knees above the hips and the shins parallel to the floor. Keep the feet relaxed. Place the arms straight up toward the ceiling with the shoulders resting wide. Lengthen the back of the neck and look straight up so the throat stays soft.

How to do it in calm steps
Breathe in through the nose and feel the ribs widen

gently toward the sides and a little toward the back. As you breathe out, tighten the imaginary seat belt around your middle by fifteen percent and keep the rib cage quiet over the pelvis. Lower the right heel toward the floor in a small arc until it lightly touches or hovers a few centimeters above the mat. Pause for a soft breath while the low back remains quiet. Breathe out again and bring the leg back to tabletop without snapping. Repeat with the left heel in the same calm manner. Continue alternating sides for the planned number of repetitions. Keep the arms reaching gently toward the ceiling and the shoulders relaxed so the neck stays free. If the lower back tries to arch or the ribs pop upward, make the arc smaller and slow the tempo.

Dose for beginners
Perform five heel taps per side for a total of ten slow repetitions. Rest for about one minute and complete a second set. If this feels heavy begin with three per side and add one each week until you reach eight to ten per side.

Progress over the weeks
Hold the pause at the bottom of the arc for one extra slow breath while the trunk stays quiet. Later extend the knee a little more as the heel travels so the lever

is longer, always within a range that keeps the ribs settled. You can also place a light miniband around the feet to add gentle resistance once the shape is steady. On days when the lower back feels sensitive, shorten the arc and keep the shins a little closer to the chest.

Common mistakes and how to correct them
Do not press the lower back aggressively into the floor or flare the ribs upward. Avoid holding the breath, shrugging the shoulders, or letting the neck strain. If these appear, reset the tabletop shape, exhale softly, think of heavy ribs and a long neck, and restart with a smaller arc.

Carryover to daily life
A trunk that stays steady while the legs move makes walking feel smoother, steadies you on stairs, and helps when you lift a light bag while turning with small steps. The back remains quiet and the hips share more of the work.

Safety notes for osteoporosis
Keep the spine neutral and avoid any fast curling or jerking. Move slowly and stay within a pain free range. If you feel sharp back pain or dizziness, stop, rest, and resume later with a smaller arc or after speaking with your clinician.

Exercise 27

Side Plank on Knees

Purpose in plain words
Build lateral trunk strength without bending the spine. This position teaches your body to resist side collapse and supports balance, walking, and lifting tasks where one side of the body works more than the other.

Equipment
Use a firm mat or carpet. A small folded towel can pad the elbow.

Starting position
Lie on your side with the forearm on the floor and the elbow directly under the shoulder. Bend both knees so the thighs point forward and the feet line up with the hips. Stack the pelvis and the rib cage so the body forms a straight line from head to knees. Place the top hand on the hip or along the side of the thigh. Keep the neck long and look straight ahead.

How to do it in calm steps
Breathe in through the nose and feel the ribs widen gently toward the sides. As you breathe out press the

forearm and the lower knee into the floor and float the pelvis upward until the body forms a straight line from head to knees. Keep the ribs quietly stacked over the pelvis and avoid pushing the chest forward. Hold the position for a slow breath while the top hip stays stacked above the bottom hip. Breathe out again as you lower the pelvis with control to return to the mat. Pause for a moment and repeat for the planned number of repetitions. Turn to the other side and perform the same sequence. If the shoulder feels pressured, slide the elbow a little farther from the body and keep the neck long.

Dose for beginners
Hold the side plank for ten to fifteen seconds per repetition. Perform four or five repetitions per side. Rest for about one minute between sides and complete two sets. If this feels heavy start with shorter holds of six to eight seconds and add a few seconds each week.

Progress over the weeks
Increase each hold to twenty seconds while keeping the same quiet ribs and long neck. Later lift the top knee a few centimeters while the feet stay together to add a gentle challenge for the side hip. Another option is to hold the top position and take three small

calm breaths before lowering. On days when the shoulder or lower back feels sensitive return to shorter holds and reduce the height of the lift.

Common mistakes and how to correct them
Do not let the pelvis roll backward or the top shoulder round forward. Avoid dropping the head toward the floor or gripping the neck. Avoid flaring the ribs or arching the lower back. If these appear lower a little, exhale softly, grow long from crown of head to knees, and imagine the space between the ribs and the floor staying open and calm.

Carryover to daily life
A steady side plank makes carrying a bag on one side, walking on uneven ground, and turning while holding a light object feel more organised. The trunk resists side sway and the spine stays protected.

Safety notes for osteoporosis
Move smoothly without jerks. Keep the spine neutral and avoid any quick twisting. If you feel sharp pain in the shoulder or back stop and resume later with a shorter hold or after adjusting the elbow position.

Exercise 28

Pallof Press with Band

Purpose in plain words
Train the trunk to resist rotation while the arms move. This builds deep support around the spine without bending or twisting and prepares you for daily tasks that try to pull your body off center.

Equipment
Use a long resistance band anchored at chest height to a solid point such as a closed door with a safe anchor or a sturdy post. Wear shoes with a grippy sole and stand on a firm surface.

Starting position
Stand side on to the anchor so the band pulls gently across your body. Hold the band with both hands at the center of your chest. Place your feet about hip width with the foot nearer the anchor slightly forward for a comfortable stance. Keep a small bend in the knees. Stack the rib cage over the pelvis so the lower back feels natural rather than arched. Let the shoulders rest wide and keep the gaze level with the horizon. Lengthen the back of the neck so the crown of the head grows tall.

How to do it in calm steps
Breathe in through the nose and allow the ribs to widen to the sides. As you breathe out, press the band straight forward from the chest until the elbows are long but not locked. Feel the band trying to pull you toward the anchor and let the trunk resist that pull without leaning. Pause for one soft breath with the hands held away from the chest. Breathe out again and bring the hands back to the chest with control while the torso stays quiet. Continue for the planned number of repetitions and keep the shoulders low and the ribs settled. Turn around to face the opposite direction so the other side of the body works equally.

Dose for beginners
Perform eight calm presses on the first side. Rest briefly and complete eight presses on the other side. Do two sets. Choose a band tension that lets you keep a smooth breath and a steady tall posture.

Progress over the weeks
Step a little farther from the anchor to increase tension or choose a slightly firmer band. Hold the arms extended for two slow breaths before returning to the chest. Later take a small step forward and back while the arms remain extended to challenge control, always keeping the spine long. On days when the

neck or lower back feels sensitive, move closer to the anchor and reduce tension so form stays crisp.

Common mistakes and how to correct them
Avoid twisting the torso toward the anchor or leaning away from it. Avoid flaring the ribs or arching the lower back. Avoid shrugging the shoulders or pushing the chin forward. If any of these appear, soften the knees, exhale gently, keep the hands at chest height, and imagine the shoulder blades sliding down and around the rib cage as you press.

Carryover to daily life
A steady anti rotation press helps when you steady a door that swings, control a dog leash, place a box on a shelf while someone bumps the table, or carry a bag on one side without swaying.

Safety notes for osteoporosis
Keep the spine neutral and the movement slow. Do not rotate quickly against the band. Inspect the anchor before each session and replace worn bands. If you feel sharp pain in the shoulders or back, stop, reset your posture, and resume only with lighter tension or after speaking with your clinician.

Exercise 29

Bird-Dog Reach Short Range

Purpose in plain words
Teach the spine to stay long while opposite arm and leg move in a small controlled range. This builds coordination and deep support for the back without forcing large arcs or fast motions.

Equipment
Use a firm mat or carpet. Wear comfortable clothing that allows the shoulders and hips to move freely.

Starting position
Begin on hands and knees with the wrists under the shoulders and the knees under the hips. Spread the fingers and press the hands gently into the floor. Keep the rib cage resting quietly over the pelvis so the lower back feels natural rather than arched. Lengthen the back of the neck and look down between your hands so the head follows the line of the spine.

How to do it in calm steps
Breathe in through the nose and feel the ribs widen gently toward the sides and a little toward the back.

As you breathe out, slide the right foot backward along the floor until the leg is long and the toes are light. At the same time slide the left hand forward along the floor so the arm is long and the fingertips are light. Pause for a soft breath while the spine stays quiet and the pelvis remains level. Breathe out again and lift the long foot and the long hand just a few centimeters from the floor, keeping the neck long and the ribs settled. Hold for one soft breath, then lower the hand and foot back to the floor and slide them into the starting position. Repeat with the left foot and the right hand in the same calm manner. Continue alternating sides for the planned number of repetitions. Keep the movement small and smooth so the back feels quiet and supported.

Dose for beginners
Perform five reaches per side for a total of ten slow repetitions. Rest for about one minute and complete a second set. If this feels heavy begin with three per side and add one each week until you reach eight to ten per side.

Progress over the weeks
Hold the lifted position for two slow breaths while the trunk stays quiet. Later extend the range slightly by lifting the hand and foot a little higher, always

within a pain free and comfortable range. You can also place a light miniband around the feet and gently press outward during the reach to engage the hips. On days when the lower back feels sensitive, keep the reach sliding on the floor without lifting and focus on the long line from fingertips to heel.

Common mistakes and how to correct them
Do not arch the lower back or let the ribs drop toward the floor. Avoid twisting the pelvis or lifting the chin. Avoid locking the elbows. If these appear, lower the limbs, exhale softly, think of length rather than height, and restart the reach with a smaller range.

Carryover to daily life
Better coordination between opposite arm and leg helps with walking on uneven ground, climbing stairs, reaching into a car seat, and steadying a light object while you turn with small steps. The spine remains protected because the trunk stays quiet.

Safety notes for osteoporosis
Move slowly and stay within a comfortable range. Keep the spine neutral and avoid fast or large motions. If you feel sharp back pain or dizziness, stop, rest, and resume later with a smaller reach or after speaking with your clinician.

Exercise 30

Tall-Kneel Hip Hinge with Dowel

Purpose in plain words
Teach the hips to hinge while the trunk stays long and quiet. The tall kneeling position removes ankle and knee distractions and lets you feel the pelvis move without arching the lower back. This pattern supports safer bending and lifting in daily life.

Equipment
Use a firm mat or folded towel for the knees. Hold a light dowel or a household broomstick. If kneeling is uncomfortable, place an extra cushion under the knees or perform the same drill in half kneel with one knee down and one foot forward.

Starting position
Kneel tall with both knees on the mat and the toes tucked under for light support, or keep the tops of the feet on the floor if that feels better. Place the dowel along your spine so one end touches the back of the head, the stick touches between the shoulder blades, and the other end touches the sacrum. Hold the dowel gently with one hand behind the neck and the other hand near the lower back so the stick maintains three

points of contact. Stack the rib cage over the pelvis and look toward the horizon so the back of the neck stays long. Engage a quiet sense of length from crown of head to knees.

How to do it in calm steps
Breathe in through the nose and allow the ribs to widen gently to the sides. As you breathe out, send the pelvis back as if you were about to sit onto an invisible stool behind you. Let the torso tip forward in one piece while all three points of the dowel remain in contact with your body. Stop when you feel a stretch in the back of the hips and the dowel still touches the head, the mid back, and the sacrum. Pause for a soft breath with the ribs settled. Breathe out again and press the shins and toes into the floor to return to tall kneel in one smooth motion without thrusting the ribs forward. Keep the shoulders relaxed and the neck long. Repeat with the same quiet rhythm, matching each effort to the exhale.

Dose for beginners
Perform eight calm repetitions. Rest for about one minute and complete a second set. If this feels heavy begin with five repetitions and add one each week until you reach ten, always keeping the stick in contact at the three points.

Progress over the weeks
Increase the hinge depth a little while the three contacts remain solid. Later hold a small backpack close to the chest and repeat the same motion, still keeping the dowel on the three points. You can also practice the movement without the dowel once the pattern is clear, and then return to the stick on days when form needs a reminder. If the knees grow tired, switch to the half kneeling version or add more padding.

Common mistakes and how to correct them
Avoid losing contact between the dowel and any of the three points. Avoid arching the lower back at the top or letting the ribs lift forward. Avoid pushing the chin ahead of the body. If these appear, slow down, exhale gently, and think of the pelvis sliding back while the head and sacrum stay connected to the stick. Keep the sense of length from crown of head to knees during the entire motion.

Carryover to daily life
A clear hip hinge in tall kneel transfers to safer bending when you reach into a low cupboard, gather a laundry basket, lift a small box, or pick up a child from a chair. The hips take the motion and the spine stays protected.

Safety notes for osteoporosis

Move slowly within a comfortable range and keep the spine neutral. Do not force deep angles or quick repetitions. If you feel knee discomfort, add padding or switch to the half kneeling setup. If you feel sharp back pain, stop and resume later with a smaller range or after speaking with your clinician.

A Small Act That Makes a Big Difference

If this book has helped you or inspired you to take better care of yourself, I have a small favor to ask: please leave a review on the platform where you purchased it. As an independent author, I don't have a big publishing house or marketing team behind me.

Every single review helps my work reach more readers and allows me to keep creating books and resources that empower others to live with strength, confidence, and peace of mind despite osteoporosis. Your words matter more than you think. A short, honest review can encourage someone who feels scared or hopeless today to believe that an active, fulfilling life is still possible.

Thank you from the heart for your support.

Elena Forti

Printed in Dunstable, United Kingdom